Smart Health Systems

Sonali Vyas • Deepshikha Bhargava

Smart Health Systems

Emerging Trends

Springer

Sonali Vyas
Department of Computer Science
University of Petroleum and Energy Studies
Dehradun, India

Deepshikha Bhargava
Department of Computer Science
University of Petroleum and Energy Studies
Dehradun, India

ISBN 978-981-16-4200-5 ISBN 978-981-16-4201-2 (eBook)
https://doi.org/10.1007/978-981-16-4201-2

This Springer imprint is published by the registered company Springer Nature Singapore Pte Ltd.
The registered company address is: 152 Beach Road, #21-01/04 Gateway East, Singapore 189721, Singapore

Contents

About the Authors

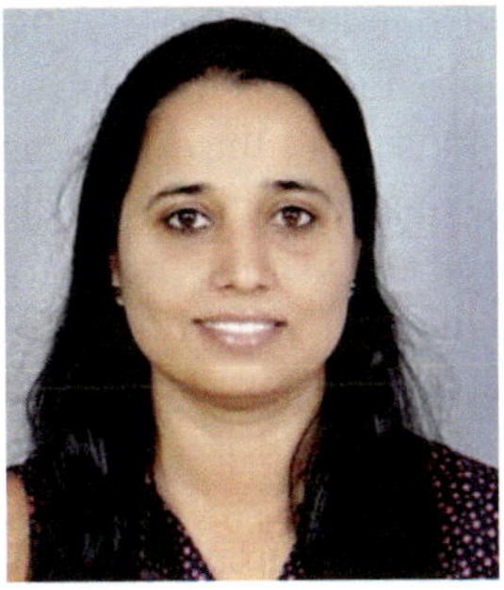

Sonali Vyas has worked as an academician and researcher for a decade. She is currently working as an assistant professor (Selection Grade) at the University of Petroleum and Energy Studies in Dehradun (Uttarakhand, India). She is a professional member of the Computer Society of India (CSI), the Institute of Electrical and Electronics Engineers (IEEE), the Association for Computing Machinery (ACM) India, the Institute For Engineering Research and Publication (IFERP), the International Association of Engineers (IAENG), the Internet Society (ISOC) and the Society for Clinical Research Sites (SCRS). She has authored numerous research papers, articles and chapters in refereed journals, conference proceedings and books. She co-edited the books *Pervasive Computing: A Networking Perspective and Future Directions*, published by Springer Nature, and *Smart Farming Technologies for Sustainable Agricultural Development*, published by IGI Global. She has acted as a guest editor for a special issue on Machine Learning and Software Systems in the *Journal of Statistics & Management Systems* (JSMS), published by Thomson Reuters. She is an editorial board member and reviewer board member for many refereed national and international journals. She has served as an active member of the organizing committees, national advisory boards and technical program committees at many national and international conferences. She has also chaired sessions at various reputed national and international conferences. In 2018, Dr Vyas received the Best Academician of the Year Award (Female) in the Global Education and Corporate Leadership (GECL) awards. In 2021 she also received "the National

Distinguished Educator Award 2021", instituted by the International Institute of organized Research (I2OR) which is a registered MSME with the Ministry of Micro, Small and Medium Enterprises, Government of India. She is also supervising PhD and M.Tech scholars in her area. Her research interest includes Data Virtualization, Data Analytics, Data Mining and Healthcare System Informatics.

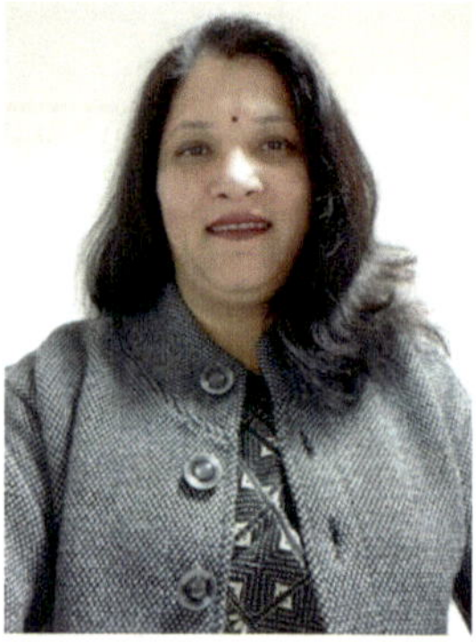

Deepshikha Bhargava has rich experience of more than 20 years as an academician. She currently works as a professor in the School of Computer Science at the University of Petroleum and Energy Studies in Dehradun (Uttarakhand, India) and is the presiding officer for the Internal Complaints Committee at the university. She previously served as a visiting professor at the Université des Mascareignes (UDM), Ministry of Education and Human Resources, Tertiary Education and Scientific Research, in Mauritius. She is a member of the Institute of Engineers (IE), the Association for Computing Machinery's Council on Women in Computing (ACM-W), the Institute of Electrical and Electronics Engineers (IEEE), the US Computer Science Teachers Association (CSTA), the Computer Society of India (CSI), the Project Management Institute (PMI), the Indian Society of Lighting Engineers (ISLE) and Vigyan Bharti (VIBHA). She has published 16 Books & 14 book chapters, edited 02 books and published 60+ research papers in journals and conference proceedings. Prof. Bhargava has previously received the Active Participation (Woman) Award and the Best Faculty of the Year award under the sub-category 'Authoring Books on Contemporary Subjects', among others. She also received an award from the Ministry of Human Resource Development (MHRD), Government of India, in 1992 for academic excellence. Overall 04 PhDs completed under her guidance. At present supervising three scholars as guide/co-guide. Her Research thrust areas are Artificial Intelligence, Soft computing, Bio-inspired computation and Healthcare informatics.

Smart Health: An Introduction

1

समदोषः समाग्निश्च समधातुमलक्रियः ।
प्रसन्नात्मेन्द्रियमनाः स्वस्थ इत्यभिधीयते । ।

Samadoshaha samaagnischa samadhaatumalakriyaha I
Prasannaatmendriyamanaaha swastha ityabhidheeyate II

Sushruta Samhita – Sutra Sthana – 15:41 (1500 BC)

In the second century BC, the *Sushruta Samhita* text offered the most comprehensive explanation of health. A similar definition of health, given by the World Health Organization (WHO) in 1948, states that:

> health is a state of complete physical, mental and social well-being and not merely an absence of disease or infirmity.

There is no doubt that health has always been considered the most important measure of our life and has a symbolic relationship with other parts of our life. A healthy body and healthy mind signify a healthy life. The emergence of technologies has influenced many parts of our daily life, including healthcare. Technological advances now underline all dimensions of healthcare, including outdoor activities, home care, in-hospital healthcare and personal healthcare, to name just a few. Information and communications technology (ICT) plays an important role in improving the quality of healthcare from traditional healthcare to smart healthcare [1].

With increases in the population, traditional healthcare now finds it difficult to provide adequate solutions for its stakeholders. The coronavirus disease 2019 (COVID-19) pandemic has now made us all even more aware of the pressures imposed on healthcare management, and these concerns are globally the same in both developed countries (such as the UK and the USA) and developing countries (such as India). Although developed countries have outstanding health frameworks

S. Vyas, D. Bhargava, *Smart Health Systems*,
https://doi.org/10.1007/978-981-16-4201-2_1

and medical facilities, and cutting-edge technologies, they are still not able to deal with such a pandemic. The situation in developing countries with large populations is much more critical.

The major issues encountered during the COVID-19 pandemic include disease prevention, creation of awareness among citizens, diagnosis of COVID-19 patients, provision of proper treatment, bed management in hospitals, the care of COVID-19 patients, prevention of coronavirus anxiety, management of healthcare services, vaccine development and distribution, and—above all—management of shortages of supplemental oxygen supplies.

The present status of traditional healthcare systems and their contributions to the COVID-19 pandemic situation give us enough reasons to replace traditional healthcare with smart healthcare.

In this chapter, readers will gain understanding of the concepts of smart health and allied areas—such as electronic health (eHealth), digital health, mobile health (mHealth), and telehealth—and the significance of each of them. The chapter concludes with a discussion of the framework and various components of smart healthcare.

1.1 What Is Smart Health?

Smart health is use of various technological advances and gadgets to provide better services for patients, hospitals, doctors and health workers. In other ways, it provides better care in the dimension of health, usually termed *smart healthcare*.

The key concepts in smart healthcare include eHealth and mHealth services, electronic record management, smart home services, and intelligent and connected medical devices.

According to Blue Stream Consultancy [1]:

> smart healthcare is defined by the technology that leads to better diagnostic tools, better treatment for patients, and devices that improve the quality of life for anyone and everyone.

The healthcare services provided by smart healthcare include [2]:

- Smart gadgets and medical wearables (such as the Fitbit and smartwatches)
- Smart healthcare products and monitoring devices (such as digital thermometers, smart glucometers and blood pressure monitors)
- The Internet of Medical Things (IoMT), wireless networks, body area networks and extensive area networks
- Smartphones and smart mobile applications (apps) for fitness, nutrition, hygiene and healthcare
- Smart devices for the elderly (hearing aids, toilet aids, walking aids, global positioning system (GPS) tracker shoe inserts etc.)
- Smart devices for persons with special needs (smart home help, smart sticks for the blind and partially sighted community, hands-free voice communication, speech to text etc.)

1.2 Objectives of Smart Healthcare

The objectives of smart healthcare are to create awareness among individuals about daily healthcare, self-checkups and health awareness, and to enable them to self-manage during medical emergencies [3].

Smart healthcare places emphasis on refining the quality and experience of healthy living for citizens and persons with special needs, including the elderly and children. It aims to ensure proper distribution, management and utilization of the available healthcare resources. Smart healthcare is not limited to any particular geographical location. It also supports remote patient monitoring, online/telemedical advice/treatment and remote surgery, among other things [4].

The main objective of smart healthcare is to provide healthcare solutions and services for daily personal and clinical healthcare. The overall objectives of smart healthcare are focused on prevention, diagnosis and treatment of disease [5].

Implementation of smart healthcare can be difficult to manage, because of data/media issues and challenges in aspects such as privacy, energy consumption, integrity, security, availability and unique identification. Figure 1.1 lists important criteria for an effective smart healthcare system with the purpose of addressing these challenges [4].

1.3 Requirements of Smart Healthcare

The objective of designing smart healthcare is to make sure appropriate medical services are provided for patients. Apart from fulfilling the basic requirements, a smart healthcare system is also aimed at improving the quality of service. The requirements of smart healthcare can be functional or nonfunctional in nature. Figure 1.2 shows the basic requirements in these two categories [4].

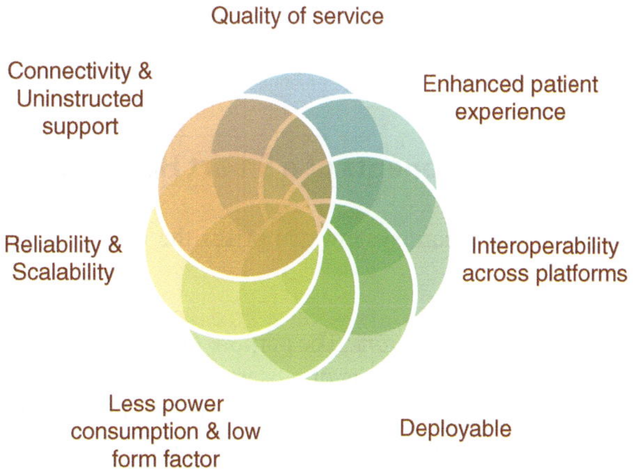

Fig. 1.1 Criteria for an effective smart healthcare system

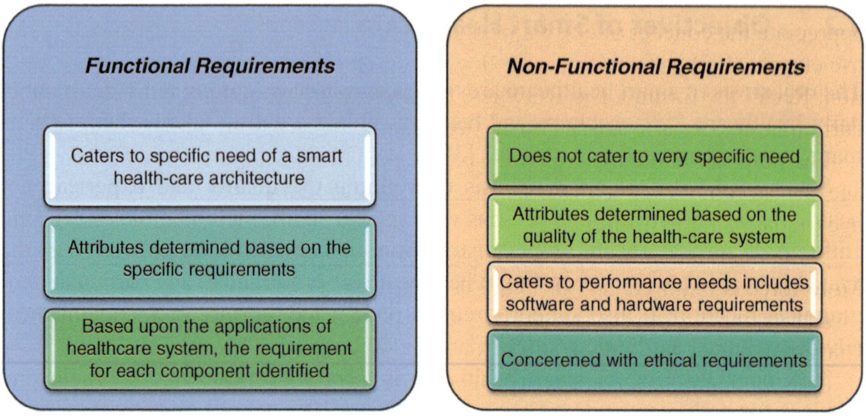

Fig. 1.2 Requirements of smart healthcare

1.4 Characteristics and Classification of Smart Healthcare

The smart healthcare system can be categorized into three broad categories, as shown in Fig. 1.3 [4]:

- *App-oriented architecture:* The characteristics of app-oriented architecture emphasize the management of applications on smartphones, including reliable and secure communication/transmission between smartphone apps, sensors, personalized networks and user devices.
- *Things-oriented architecture:* The purpose of things-oriented architecture is to ensure real-time monitoring of the delivery and efficiency of applications.
- *Semantics-oriented architecture:* Semantics-oriented architecture is aimed at a better user experience based on behavioural patterns and acquired information.

In addition, smart healthcare involves heterogeneous and location-aware computing, impulsive collaboration, and use of dynamic and distributed networks with higher efficiency.

1.5 Components of a Smart Healthcare System

A smart healthcare system comprises the following four components, as shown in Fig. 1.4 [4]:

- *Sensors and actuators:* The purpose of an Internet of Things (IoT)–based sensor is to measure the vital signs of a user/patient. Sensors/actuators include sensors to measure the body temperature, cardiac signals, blood pressure, blood glucose, heart rate, oxygen saturation, and speed and motion of the patients, to name just a few.

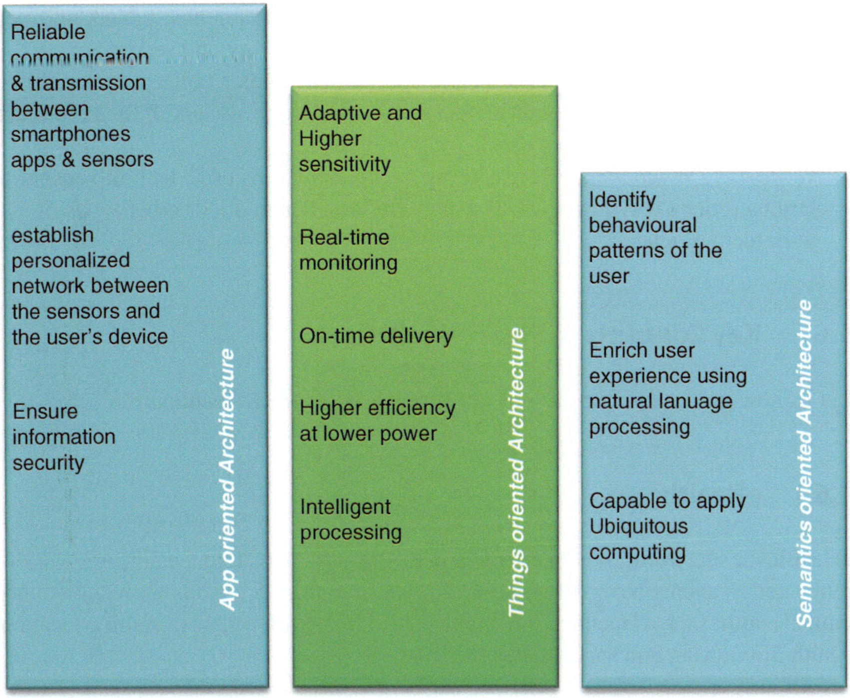

Fig. 1.3 Characteristics of smart healthcare

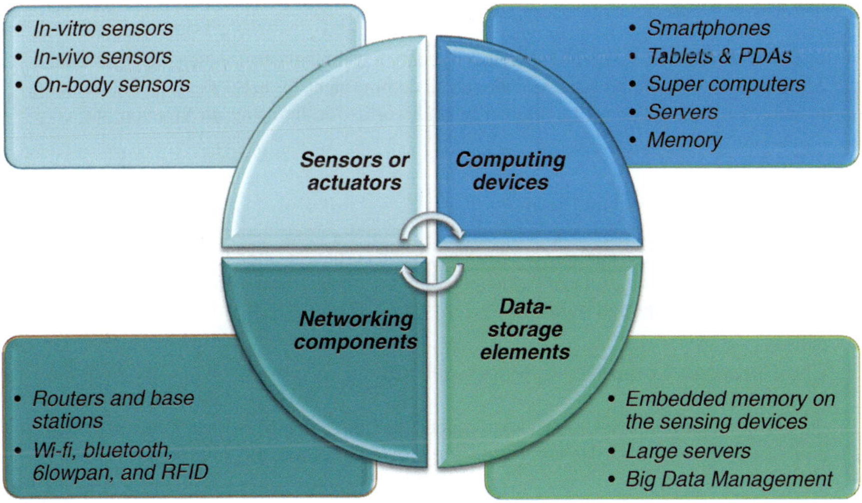

Fig. 1.4 Components of smart healthcare

- *Computing devices:* Computing devices include smartphones, tablets and personal digital assistants (PDAs), supercomputers, memory and servers.
- *Data storage components:* The health and vital signs data collected from different sensors are stored in embedded memory and large servers in the cloud, and they are analysed using big data.
- *Networking components:* Networking components are used to link sensors to various routers and base stations using wireless, Bluetooth or other types of network technologies.

1.6 Key Concepts in Smart Healthcare

Let us now go through the various key terms used in smart healthcare.

1.6.1 eHealth

eHealth, or electronic health, is related to the use of ICT in healthcare. Various renowned agencies have defined eHealth and mentioned various terms associated with eHealth, such as medical informatics, healthcare informatics, health education, health monitoring and surveillance [6].

The *Journal of Medical Internet Research* defines eHealth as:

> an emerging field in the intersection of medical informatics, public health and business, referring to health services and information delivered or enhanced through the Internet and related technologies.
>
> In a broader sense, the term characterizes not only a technical development, but also a state-of-mind, a way of thinking, an attitude, and a commitment for networked, global thinking, to improve healthcare locally, regionally, and worldwide by using information and communication technology.

The WHO defines eHealth as:

> the cost-effective and secure use of information and communication technologies in support of the health and health-related fields including healthcare, health surveillance and health education, knowledge and research.

The European Commission defines eHealth as:

> the use of modern information and communication technologies to meet needs of citizens, patients, healthcare professionals, healthcare providers, as well as policy makers.

The objectives of eHealth are to provide health literacy, support better communication among all healthcare stakeholders (hospitals, patients, researchers, physicians, health workers and health insurance companies), assist healthcare and hospital management, and assist disease prevention and well-being monitoring. Examples of eHealth are electronic health records (EHRs)[1], telemedicine and health portals [7].

1.6.2 Digital Health

Digital health involves use of digital care services and varied technologies to address healthcare challenges by adapting medicine to ubiquitous ICTs. Digital Health encompasses the use of digital tools to provide better healthcare and better patient experiences, and support for medical professionals in medicine and healthcare. The objective of digital health is to connect all stakeholders in healthcare through digital channels [7]. Digital health includes all services and devices for personal healthcare, such as smart apps, wearable devices, augmented and virtual reality, assistive technologies for the elderly and persons with special needs, electronic medical records (EMRs), smart gadgets and smart homes.

Traditionally, the terms *eHealth* and *digital health* have been used interchangeably; however, these terms differ on the following bases:

- eHealth is aimed at improving quality and knowledge in healthcare, using ICT, whereas digital health is aimed at implementation of ICT to address healthcare challenges.
- eHealth tools include products, systems and frameworks, whereas digital health is related to services for personal healthcare and well-being.

1.6.3 mHealth

mHealth refers to mobile health and includes the practices of medicine and public health with the help of mobile devices such as smartphones, tablets and PDAs, and wireless setups. mHealth comprises telecommunications and multimedia technologies for dissemination of health information and healthcare management. Examples of mHealth are mobile applications for healthcare education and awareness, disease diagnosis and treatment, dissemination of healthcare information through a short message service (SMS), smart alert systems, emergency response systems, decision support systems for physicians and the point of care, patient safety systems, healthcare supply chains, remote healthcare and telemedicine, to name a few. Overall, mHealth is aimed at improving quality and convenience, and reducing healthcare costs for patients [8].

[1] An electronic health record (EHR) is a digital summary of a patient's entire medical history and is designed to be shared by multiple healthcare providers. It differs from an electronic medical record (EMR), which is a digital record of a patient's chart used by a single healthcare provider.

1.6.4 Smart Health IT

Smart Health IT is an open standards–based technology platform to transform EHRs into platforms for substitutable iPhone-like apps. It provides a facility of universal application programming interfaces (APIs) to create apps for secure healthcare systems and offers a library of apps to improve clinical care, research and development (R&D) and public health [9].

1.6.5 Smart Hospitals

Smart hospitals are a smarter way of treating and healing patients by reducing patient waiting time, improving the quality of patient care, lowering infection risks, optimizing staff productivity, providing health data management and data warehousing, enhancing patients' experiences and satisfaction, reducing errors in patient management and providing rapid emergency responses [10].

In the present scenario of the COVID-19 pandemic and the consequent pressure on hospitals, there is an urgent need for future-ready smart hospitals to address the healthcare challenges faced by hospitals and help them adjust to the "new normal".

The objectives of smart hospitals are not only to enhance patients' experiences by use of emerging smart technologies in their design but also to develop a healthcare delivery ecosystem in which hospitals are connected with stakeholders and governments. The key reasons behind the reshaping of global healthcare ecosystems and the requirement for smart hospitals are focuses on value, accountability, quality, outcome-based clinical research, health management (instead of only disease treatment), independent health services without physical boundaries and the increasing number of informed patients [11].

1.7 Concluding Remarks

This chapter has presented an overview of the basic concept of smart health and its characteristics, requirements, classification and components. The chapter has also highlighted various key terms that the reader needs to know.

After reading this chapter, the reader will be able to define smart health, smart healthcare and various components of a smart healthcare system.

Keeping in view the pandemic situation across the globe, the chapter has also presented the need for analysis of smart health and smart hospitals.

The chapter has discussed technologies and devices only in brief. The technologies used in smart healthcare are explored further in Chap. 2.

References

1. Active Advice (2017) What is smart health and how do people benefit? https://www.activeadvice.eu/news/concept-projects/what-is-smart-health-and-how-do-people-benefit/. Accessed on 20/12/2020
2. Ahad A, Tahir M, Yau K-LA (2019) 5G-based smart healthcare network: architecture, taxonomy, challenges and future research directions. IEEE Access 7:100747–100762. https://doi.org/10.1109/ACCESS.2019.2930628
3. Mohanty SP, Choppali U, Kougianos E (2016) Everything you wanted to know about smart cities: the Internet of Things is the backbone. IEEE Consum Electron Mag 5(3):60–70
4. Sundaravadivel P, Kougianos E, Mohanty SP, Ganapathiraju MK (2017) Evaluating the different technologies and components of the Internet of Things for better health. IEEE Consum Electron Mag 7(1):18–28. https://doi.org/10.1109/MCE.2017.2755378
5. Yin H, Akmandor AO, Mosenia A, Jha NK (2018) Smart healthcare. Found Trends Electron Des Autom 12(4):401–466. https://doi.org/10.1561/1000000054
6. Innovatemedtec (2021) eHealth. https://innovatemedtec.com/digital-health/ehealth. Accessed on 26/4/2021
7. Khillar S (2020) Difference between eHealth and digital health. Difference between.net. http://www.differencebetween.net/technology/difference-between-ehealth-and-digital-health/. Accessed 15/3/2021
8. Innovatemedtec (2021) mHealth. https://innovatemedtec.com/digital-health/mhealth. Accessed 18/5/2021
9. SmartHealthIT (2019) Smart®. https://smarthealthit.org/. Accessed 15/2/2021
10. Siemens (2021) Smart hospitals. https://new.siemens.com/global/en/markets/healthcare/smart-hospitals.html. Accessed 12/6/2021
11. Chen B, Baur A, Stepniak M, Wang J (2019) Finding the future of care provision: the role of smart hospitals. McKinsey & Company. https://www.mckinsey.com/industries/healthcare-systems-and-services/our-insights/finding-the-future-of-care-provision-the-role-of-smart-hospitals. Accessed 20/2/2021

2 Technologies for Smart Health

Chapter 1 discussed the basic concepts of smart health and allied areas such as eHealth, digital health, mHealth, telehealth, and various components of smart healthcare.

Now, we will move ahead and try to understand the technologies that can be used to develop solutions for all participants in smart healthcare, such as physicians, patients, hospitals and researchers [1].

This chapter focuses first on the impacts of technologies on smart healthcare. Subsequent sections discuss next-generation technologies for smart healthcare (and examples of them), and smart healthcare applications and products [2]. The chapter concludes with the positive and negative impacts of technology on healthcare.

2.1 Impacts of Technologies on Smart Healthcare

The advent of technologies such as cloud computing, big data, blockchains, artificial intelligence (AI), fifth-generation cellular wireless networks (5G networks) etc. has had multifaceted impacts on society, including the medical industry and healthcare. In healthcare, these technologies exemplify changes in patient care, medical innovations, personal care, remote consultation, diagnosis and clinical trials. The major focus of technology has shifted towards preventive healthcare and the patient experience, along with disease treatment [3].

Technology has impacted various dimensions ranging from personal healthcare to preventive healthcare. This impact can be realized with the development of smart wearables; remote surgery; virtual medical assistants; remote home services; intelligent clinical systems for diagnosis, research, clinical trials and decision-making; electronic medical records (EMRs) and electronic health records (EHRs); and drug discovery, management and screening [2].

Optimization of the impacts of technologies for smart healthcare depends on appropriate utilization of medical resources, minimization of the costs and risk of

S. Vyas, D. Bhargava, *Smart Health Systems*,
https://doi.org/10.1007/978-981-16-4201-2_2

medical procedures, provision of remote accessibility irrespective of the geographical location, and encouragement of pervasive and personalized healthcare [2].

Technology has brought a welcome transformation to healthcare and provided significant assistance to patients, doctors, hospitals, pharmacists, nurses and other healthcare workers in both general and emergency situations. For example, online consultations and telemedicine connect medical professionals to patients and provide a facility for basic treatments; they also connect hospitals and pharmacists to patients [4].

2.2 Next-Generation Technologies for Smart Healthcare

Everyone wants to be healthy and hopes they will not need to visit a hospital; however, it is sometimes necessary to do so, including visits for regular medical fitness checkups. Usually, the hospital environment is stressful for visitors, whether they are patients or caregivers. The processes used in traditional hospitals are usually cumbersome, whether a visitor is attending an appointment with a physician, undergoing medical examinations, or collecting medical reports.

The coronavirus disease 2019 (COVID-19) pandemic situation has hugely increased these stresses across the world. In an emergency situation such as a pandemic, hospitals, doctors and healthcare workers are overstressed because of the massive and critical patient loads. In both normal and "new normal" conditions, it is necessary not only to provide solutions to the limitations of the traditional hospital system but also to address the need for personalized healthcare. Smart healthcare products and services can address such challenges [5].

Next-generation technologies such as cloud computing, big data, blockchains, mobile technology, the Internet of Things (IoT), AI and 5G networks enable smart healthcare systems to be manageable and functional. Let us now go through the role of each of these technologies in smart healthcare (Fig. 2.1).

2.2.1 RFID Technology

Radiofrequency identification (RFID) technology uses radiofrequency devices and a suitable setup to store and retrieve massive volumes of data, using wireless/electromagnetic transmission [6, 7].

Barcoding is used in hospitals, but, because of its technical limitations, RFID technology has been considered as an alternative approach to manage and improve functional efficacy in hospitals [8, 9]. RFID-based solutions can be used effectively to save staff time spent in real-time tracing and location of inventory items, medical devices and patients; identify appropriate utilization of medical resources; minimize medical errors in clinical examinations; manage medical/clinical requirements; and perform security and surveillance functions [7, 10, 11]. RFID technology can also be used to improve the efficiency of patient care in terms of recording/reporting of vital signs, use of medical aids/devices, and communications [4]. Thus, RFID

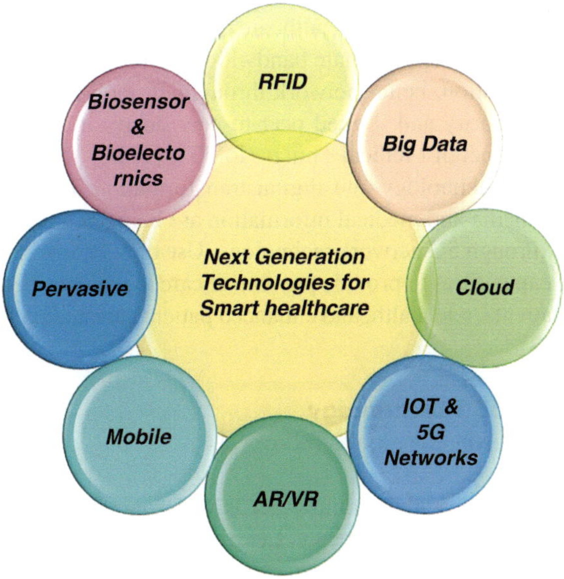

Fig. 2.1 Next-generation technologies for smart healthcare

technology provides suitable support for hospital inventory management, as well as patient care.

2.2.2 IoT Technology and 5G Networks

Smart healthcare systems are aimed at transformation of a conventional hospital-focused approach into a distributed patient-focused approach. At present, smart healthcare services and applications are based on 4G networks; however, 4G networks are not able to deal with massive volumes of data (i.e. big data produced/used in smart healthcare systems or IoT healthcare products) and have limited capabilities in terms of bandwidth, latency and peer-to-peer delay.

For example, patients who need medical advice currently need to visit hospitals/clinics, which might be convenient in urban areas but is a challenge in rural areas. With the advent of remote consultation and telehealth, this challenge can be overcome. However, at the same time, there may be challenges in ensuring network connectivity to enable video conferencing, uploading/downloading of medical prescriptions, remote monitoring and medical imaging, to name just a few requirements.

Similar challenges have been witnessed in emergency situations (e.g. the need for medical aid during the Kedarnath disaster in India and the COVID-19 pandemic worldwide) requiring remote communications in rural areas to assist delivery of medical care to patients. In such situations, the major challenges have been related to establishment of networks/communications, remote communications, slow network speeds, patient monitoring, unnecessary delays etc.

To address such limitations, 5G networks are considered the best approach for IoT-based diverse and time-critical healthcare applications. Moreover, 5G network–enabled technology provides adequate bandwidth, energy efficiency, better connectivity and communication, better network throughput, mobile coverage, minimum time complexity, security and limited peer-to-peer delays in networks of medical devices (i.e. the Internet of Medical Things (IoMT)) [12].

With use of IoT technology and digital transformation in healthcare, massive amounts of multimedia and medical information are being generated, which can be easily managed through 5G network technology. Use of 5G networks with IoT technology enables capabilities to provide preventive care to patients, better remote connectivity with patients, telehealth, and enhanced patient care and patient experiences at lower costs [13].

2.2.2.1 Impacts of 5G Technology

The impacts of 5G technology are as follows [14]:

- 5G technology can provide ultrafast speeds with low latency for telehealth and remote support for quality healthcare. Let us consider the upsurge in the coronavirus pandemic, wherein 5G networks can provide remote consultations for COVID-19 patients to reduce exposure to the contagion. This approach can also provide immediate medical support and treatment for critically ill patients or patients in quarantine/home isolation.
- 5G networks can also assist traditional hospitals to transform into smart hospitals. According to AT&T, "adding a high-speed 5G network to existing architectures can help quickly and reliably transport huge data files of medical imagery, which can improve both access to care and the quality of care. At the Austin Cancer Centre, the PET [positron emission tomography] scanner generates extremely large files—up to 1 gigabyte of information per patient per study."
- Massive amounts of medical/patient information can be uploaded/downloaded at faster speeds.
- Timely prevention, diagnostics, remote monitoring and treatment can be provided for patients.
- In comparison with fibre-based networks, 5G networks have the potential to provide greater network bandwidths and speeds for transmission of medical imaging and diagnostic data.
- 5G technology can provide adequate support for the emergence and use of wearable devices.

2.2.3 Big Data

As was noted in the previous section, massive volumes of data are generated through use of IoT technology in healthcare. There is therefore a need to address issues related to storage, analytics and predictive analytics. Use of big data in healthcare addresses such data storage and management-related requirements [4].

Big data technology can be used in healthcare to describe, store and manage huge volumes of health and medical data generation with digital transformation (e.g. data related to patients' vital signs, medical device inventories in hospitals and clinical data). The same data can also be used for analytics and generation of predictions, using a big data analysis approach [15].

Overall, big data technology provides adequate support for improvement of predictions related to patients and disease; medical imaging; real-time alerts, self-harm prevention, risk/fraud and disease management; smart staffing and strategic planning for optimal work time utilization; optimization of EHRs and electronic medication records; telemedicine; enhanced patient satisfaction and experience; and, above all, medical research (including clinical trials) and disease diagnosis [15].

The different types of big data include clinical trial data, EHRs, administrative data, claims data, patient/disease registries and health surveys [16].

2.2.4 The Cloud

As we have seen, storage and management of big data are important measures in healthcare. At the same time, the choice of storage media is equally important. Physical storage means (hard disks, compact disks (CDs), portable drives etc.) have limited storage capabilities. For remote healthcare options, storage of data on physical media has limited capabilities. Hence, there is a requirement to store such data in a medium that is accessible, secure, cost effective, portable, reliable and efficient. The solution is cloud storage, which addresses the storage and management requirements and backup/recovery requirements related to health data. In addition, cloud services are available for effective research and analysis on medical data [4].

2.2.5 Augmented Reality/Virtual Reality

Human brains find it easier to process data when it is presented in a visual form. With the advent of digital transformation, augmented and virtual reality (AR/VR) offer new dimensions for visual display of data and analytics. VR devices and applications provide a platform to showcase and analyse patient vital signs, disease, mood management, anxiety/stress management, fitness and patient recovery. At the same time, AR applications and devices can support physicians/surgeons performing remote surgery, disease diagnosis, gene therapy, gene analytics and protein synthesis, to name just a few possibilities [4].

2.2.6 Mobile Technologies

Mobile technologies for healthcare include computers on wheels (COWs), workstations on wheels (WOWs), blood donation mobile vans, mobile testing, smart ambulances and, above all, mobile applications (apps).

Smartphones are the gadgets that are most commonly used by all of us. Among the smart features provided by smartphones, mobile apps are the most frequently used and popular ones. Healthcare mobile apps have been identified as preferred choices for downloading and 24/7 use. The variety of health apps available cover such aspects as health and fitness, sleep management, stress management, medical records, appointments, clinical decision-making, clinical reports, medicine notifications, healthy diet and nutrition plans, personal care, and drug information for improved diagnosis [4].

According to Liquid-State, "in 2018 there were over 318,000 mobile healthcare apps available for patients, and approximately 200 new healthcare apps being built each day. This number is staggering, and we can assume that this number has increased substantially since the COVID-19 pandemic" [17].

According to Brian Kalis, the managing director of digital health and innovation for Accenture's health business, "simply having a mobile app is not enough.... Apps are failing to engage patients by not aligning their functionality and user experience with what consumers expect and need. Consumers want ubiquitous access to products and services as part of their customer experience, and those who become disillusioned with a provider's mobile services—or a lack thereof—could look elsewhere for services" [17].

Let us now take a brief look at some popular mobile apps for healthcare [17–20].

Mobile apps for use by healthcare providers include the following:

- AHRQ ePSS—screening and prevention tool
- Archimedes—medical calculator
- Box—cloud storage and file sharing
- Calculate—medical calculator
- Diagnosaurus—differential diagnosis
- Doximity—social networking for medical professionals
- Dropbox—cloud storage and file sharing
- Dynamed—drug and medical reference
- Epocrates—drug and medical reference
- Evernote—note-taking and organization
- Gauss Pixel—measurement of the amount of blood loss in surgical procedures
- GoodReader—PDF viewer
- Google Drive—cloud storage and file sharing
- iAnnotate—PDF viewer
- Lab Pro Values—laboratory reference
- Leafly—for the cannabis community
- MDacne—custom acne treatment
- MedPage Today—medical news
- Medscape—medical reference
- Micromedex—drug reference
- Notability—note-taking and organization
- QuantiaMD—continuing medical education
- Skyscape/Omnio—drug and medical reference

Mobile apps for patient monitoring include the following:

- AirStrip One—EMRs
- Lab Pro Values—laboratory reference
- MedCalc—medical calculator
- Mediquations—medical calculator
- Pocket Lab Values—laboratory reference

Mobile apps for personal healthcare include the following:

- Diabetes Manager by WellDoc
- MySugr—diabetes tracker log
- Welch Allyn iExaminer Adapter and Ophthalmoscope—retinal detachment or glaucoma

Mobile apps for medical imaging include the following:

- AliveCor—cardiac measurements
- Mobile MIM—to share images from radiation oncology, radiology, nuclear medicine, neuroimaging and cardiac imaging
- ResolutionMD
- Visual DX—cancer prediction

Mobile apps for online consultation include the following:

- 5-Minute Clinical Consult (5MCC)—clinical consultation
- 5-Minute Infectious Diseases Consult (5MIDC)—clinical consultation
- Better Help—online counselling
- ClotMD—anticoagulant medication
- ePocrates ID—clinical consultation
- EyeCare Live
- Heal—remote physician consultation
- IDdx—clinical consultation
- Infectious Disease Notes (ID Notes)—clinical consultation
- Johns Hopkins Antibiotic Guide (JHABx)—clinical consultation
- Medici
- MyChart
- Pocket Medicine Infectious Diseases (PMID)—clinical consultation
- Sanford Guide to Antimicrobial Therapy (SG)—clinical consultation
- Teladoc—24/7 access to a doctor
- UpToDate—clinical consultation

Mobile apps for wellness include the following:

- Clue—mood analysis
- Exhale—stress reduction, relaxation and meditation

- Generis—DNA and nutrition
- Headspace—meditation
- Healthifyme—Diet, sports and fitness activity tracking
- Maya—menstrual period tracking
- Mindset—sleep cycle analysis
- Noom—diet and nutrition
- [Pharmacy apps]
- [Pregnancy apps]
- [Weight loss coaching apps]

2.2.7 Pervasive and Personalized Healthcare

The concept of pervasive healthcare refers to 24/7 availability of healthcare to everyone remotely, irrespective of their geographical location. It includes regular and periodic health checkups, healthcare monitoring, disease prevention, diagnosis and treatment [21].

2.2.8 Biosensors and Bioelectronics on Smartphones

Along with the extensive use of mobile apps on smartphones, it is possible to use sensors and sensor data collected via smartphones for healthcare purposes. For example, accelerometer and gyrometer functions can be used in fitness applications, handheld detectors can be used in real-time monitoring and biometric sensors can be used for personal checkups [22].

2.3 Smart Healthcare Applications and Products

2.3.1 Assistance with Diagnosis and Treatment

With application of AI, various healthcare solutions can be provided to assist in diagnosis and treatment, such as surgical robots, AR/VR for surgical planning, clinical support systems for management of General diseases to Critical cases and smart radiomics for remote monitoring of patient radiotherapy.

2.3.2 Health Management

Health management includes patient self-care, use of smart wearable devices and gadgets, smart homes, smart health information systems (HISs), real-time self-monitoring of patients, instant response of health data, and well-timed medical interventions.

2.3.3 Disease Prevention and Risk Monitoring

Disease risk prediction and monitoring systems accumulate data from smart wearables and mobile apps, upload them to the cloud through a 5G network and evaluate the results, using big data for predictive analytics.

2.3.4 Virtual Assistants

Virtual assistants provide assistance to patients and doctors for remote communication. They includes natural language processing, speech recognition, speech-to-text etc. Virtual assistants can be classified as conversational assistants and social-based medical virtual assistants.

2.3.5 Smart Hospitals, Rooms and Homes

Smart hospitals integrate multiple digital systems based on IoT devices, intelligent buildings and personnel. This technology can also be used for patient identification and monitoring, staff management and tracking of health inventories or specimens.

Smart rooms and smart homes use sensors/actuators to provide home assistance for elderly and disabled patients, with home automation and health monitoring. They are like having a smart hospital at home.

2.3.6 Assistance with Drug Research

This technology provides assistance with drug development, target screening, drug discovery and clinical trials.

2.3.7 Telemedicine/Telehealth

Telemedicine addresses challenges related to location barriers and critical care in emergency situations, and also supports home care [4].

2.4 Positive and Negative Effects of Technology

Positive effects of technology use include the following [23, 24]:

- Enhanced learning experiences using smart apps, smart boards, document cameras, Apple TVs, and even three-dimensional (3D) printers to incorporate collaboration and project-based learning

- Research and development
- Facilitation of fitness and health
- Opportunities for remote consultation
- Management of personal healthcare and mental health
- Provision of pervasive healthcare
- Support for hospital management
- Enhancement of medical data management
- Enhancement of diagnosis and treatment
- Support for clinical trials
- Improved patient experiences

Negative effects of technology use include the following [23, 24].

- Issues related to integrity and security of critical health data and patient vital sign data
- Negative impacts on eyesight and hearing capabilities, due to overuse of mobile apps
- Unnecessary anxiety due to excessive real-time monitoring of health data
- Absence of the rewarding social connections normally associated with meetings in person
- Stimulation of health issues such as obesity, unhealthy habits and poor sleep management

References

1. Farahani B, Firouzi F, Chang V, Badaroglu M, Constant N, Mankodiya K (2018) Towards fog-driven IoT eHealth: promises and challenges of loT in medicine and healthcare. Futur Gener Comput Syst 78(Pt 2):659–676
2. Tian S, Yang W, Le Grange JM, Wang P, Huang W, Ye Z (2019) Smart healthcare: making medical care more intelligent. Global Health J 3(3):62–65. https://doi.org/10.1016/j.glohj.2019.07.001
3. Liu BH, He KL, Zhi G (2018) The impact of big data and artificial intelligence on the future medical model. J Life Environ Sci 39(22):1–4
4. Jones M (2018) Healthcare: how technology impacts the healthcare industry. Healthcare in America. https://healthcareinamerica.us/healthcare-how-technology-impacts-the-healthcare-industry-b2ba6271c4b4. Accessed on 28/5/2021
5. Sundaravadivel P, Kougianos E, Mohanty SP, Ganapathiraju MK (2018) Everything you wanted to know about smart health care: evaluating the different technologies and components of the Internet of Things for better health. IEEE Consum Electron Mag 7(1):18–28. https://doi.org/10.1109/MCE.2017.2755378
6. Seol S, Lee EK, Kim W (2017) Indoor mobile object tracking using RFID. Futur Gener Comput Syst 76:443–451
7. Yazici HJ (2014) An exploratory analysis of hospital perspectives on real time information requirements and perceived benefits of RFID technology for future adoption. Int J Inf Manag 34(5):603–621

8. Coustasse A, Tomblin S, Slack C (2013) Impact of radio-frequency identification (RFID) technologies on the hospital supply chain: a literature review. Perspect Health Inf Manag 10:1
9. Chan HL, Choi TM, Hui CL (2012) RFID versus bar-coding systems: transactions errors in health care apparel inventory control. Decis Support Syst 54(1):803–811
10. Camacho-Cogollo JE, Bonet I, Iadanza E (2020) Chapter 4: RFID technology in health care. In: Iadanza E (ed) Clinical engineering handbook, 2nd edn. Academic, London, pp 33–41. https://doi.org/10.1016/B978-0-12-813467-2.00004-3
11. Wamba SF, Anand A, Carter L (2013) A literature review of RFID-enabled healthcare applications and issues. Int J Inf Manag 33(5):875–891
12. Ahad A, Tahir M, Aman Sheikh M, Ahmed KI, Mughees A, Numani A (2020) Technologies trend towards 5G network for smart health-care using IoT: a review. Sensors (Basel) 20(14):4047. https://doi.org/10.3390/s20144047
13. AT&T Business (2021) 5 ways 5G will transform healthcare: improving patient experience with personalized, preventative care. https://www.business.att.com/learn/updates/how-5gwill-transform-the-healthcare-industry.html. Accessed on 16/5/2021
14. Stracuzzi M (2020) 4 revolutionary use cases of 5G in healthcare. Telit. https://www.telit.com/blog/4-revolutionary-use-cases-5g-healthcare/. Accessed on 15/5/2021
15. Durcevic S (2020) 18 examples of big data analytics in healthcare that can save people. Datapine. https://www.datapine.com/blog/big-data-examples-in-healthcare/. Accessed on 16/5/2021
16. Health Sciences Library (2021) Data resources in the health sciences. University of Washington. https://guides.lib.uw.edu/hsl/data/findclin. Accessed on 16/4/2021
17. Fajardo A (2021) 8 best healthcare apps for patients|top mobile apps in 2021. Rootstrap. https://www.rootstrap.com/blog/healthcare-apps/. Accessed on 15/5/2021
18. Ventola CL (2014) Mobile devices and apps for health care professionals: uses and benefits. Pharm Ther 39(5):356–364
19. Continuum (2021) 7 best FDA approved health apps. https://www.carecloud.com/continuum/7-best-fda-approved-health-apps/. Accessed on 16/5/2021
20. Sagar P (2020) 5 most innovative healthcare apps of 2020. Electronic Health Reporter. https://electronichealthreporter.com/5-most-innovative-healthcare-apps-of-2020/. Accessed on 20/5/2021
21. Varshney U (2005) Pervasive healthcare: applications, challenges and wireless solutions. Commun Assoc Inf Syst 16(3):57–72. https://doi.org/10.17705/1CAIS.01603
22. Zhang D, Liu Q (2016) Biosensors and bioelectronics on smartphone for portable biochemical detection. Biosens Bioelectron 75:273–284. https://doi.org/10.1016/j.bios.2015.08.037
23. Stueber S (2019) The positive and negative effects of technology on children. West Bend. https://www.thesilverlining.com/westbendcares/blog/the-positive-and-negative-effects-of-technology-on-children. Accessed on 14/5/2021
24. Pajama Jack (2021) The good and bad impact of technology on health. https://panamajack.com/blogs/tips-n-tricks/the-good-and-bad-impact-of-technology-on-health. Accessed on 10/5/2021

3 Telehealth

This chapter discusses the different concepts of telecare, telehealth and telemedicine. The chapter begins with the basic concepts of telehealth; its goals, issues, needs and trends. It then discusses the differences between telehealth and telemedicine, provides examples, and discusses common uses and mobile applications (apps) for telemedicine and telehealth. The chapter concludes with the technical requirements of a telehealth app, a guide for setting up such an app, and the pros and cons of telemedicine.

3.1 What Is Telehealth?

Telehealth refers to remote healthcare services aimed at improving or managing healthcare, using information and communications technology (ICT), mobile devices and computing devices [1].

The World Health Organization (WHO) defines telehealth as [2]:

> the delivery of health care services, where distance is a critical factor, by all health care professionals using information and communication technologies for the exchange of valid information for diagnosis, treatment and prevention of disease and injuries, research and evaluation, and for the continuing education of health care providers, all in the interests of advancing the health of individuals and their communities.

According to the American Telemedicine Association (ATA) [2]:

> telemedicine is the use of medical information exchanged from one site to another via electronic communications to improve a patient's clinical health status. Telemedicine includes a growing variety of applications and services using two-way video, email, smart phones, wireless tools and other forms of telecommunications technology.

It can therefore be understood that telehealth can be used for personal and pervasive healthcare at home, using various means such as smartphones to upload data on

S. Vyas, D. Bhargava, *Smart Health Systems*,
https://doi.org/10.1007/978-981-16-4201-2_3

vital signs, food logs and medication dosing; assess health conditions by watching various relevant videos or apps; understand diet and nutrition requirements; follow healthy plans for fitness and mental wellbeing; view appointments, prescriptions, electronic medical records (EMRs) and clinical test results online; and use reminders via email/short message service (SMS) for preventive care such as vaccinations [1]. Telehealth is also sometimes referred to as eHealth or mHealth.

The US Health Resources Services Administration (HRSA) [2] defines telehealth as:

> the use of electronic information and telecommunications technologies to support long-distance clinical health care, patient and professional health-related education, public health and health administration. Technologies include videoconferencing, the internet, store-and-forward imaging, streaming media, and terrestrial and wireless communications.

According to the US Centers for Medicare and Medicaid Services (CMS) and the US Federation of State Medical Boards (FSMB) [2], telemedicine provides real-time, remote, electronic and interactive/two-way communication over audio/video/telephone/email/instant messaging between patients and medical practitioners.

3.2 The Needs and Goals of Telehealth

Let us consider the current status of traditional healthcare services. Traditional healthcare offers only limited medical services to patients in distant locations and rural areas. This provides valid reasons to use telehealth services; however, it involves a few requirements such as network coverage and payment, licensing of medical professionals, authorization and privilege, remote medical counselling, procedures for addressing misconduct and professional liability, privacy and security, and avoidance of fraud and abuse. Furthermore, it is necessary to provide adequate network connectivity and to conduct proper research to evaluate telehealth from time to time and ensure that it is a value-based delivery system for healthcare [3].

To address the basic needs of the healthcare service, the main goal of telehealth is to ensure interactive and remote communication among all healthcare stakeholders, using ICT tools. The major goals of telehealth are [1]:

- To provide healthcare that is reachable irrespective of the users' geographical locations, including rural and or isolated populations
- To provide healthcare services that are handily available for people with immobility and time constraints
- To be responsible for accessibility of healthcare workers and medical practitioners
- To establish adequate, interactive and uninterrupted communication between all users
- To provide support for personal healthcare and self-care

3.3 Telemedicine Trends

Let us now look at the trends in the history of the telemedicine industry. It was previously reported by Mordor Intelligence [4] that telemedicine would be worth more than US$66 billion by the year 2021 and that, in combination with telehealth, it could reach a value of US$175.5 billion by 2026. CB Insights reported record levels of financing in telehealth in the first quarter of 2020: with patients increasingly turning to online doctor visits, telemedicine funding almost tripled in comparison with the fourth quarter of 2019. The coronavirus disease 2019 (COVID-19) pandemic has already transformed the healthcare services landscape drastically [5].

Telemedicine is inclusive and covers all ages, underprivileged people, patients with chronic diseases, and other susceptible groups of people who depend on it.

3.4 Issues Related to Telehealth

On the basis of these market trends, telemedicine needs to address the following issues [3, 6]:

- The needs for better coverage, connectivity, technology and accessibility of telehealth apps for all users
- The rise in distributed healthcare and flexibility
- The needs to ensure security and privacy to prevent fraud and cyberattacks, given the complete dependence of telemedicine on ICT
- The need to provide support for allied areas of telemedicine
- The need for a secure third-party platform for the telemedicine industry
- The requirement for a needs-based facility to reach hospitals
- The need to ensure that the right care is available in the right place at the right time
- The need to overcome barriers to adoption of telehealth
- The need for opportunities for private players to participate in telehealth services

3.5 Differences Between Telemedicine, Telecare and Telehealth

According to the HRSA [2]:

> telehealth is different from telemedicine because it refers to a broader scope of remote healthcare services than telemedicine. While telemedicine refers specifically to remote clinical services, telehealth can refer to remote non-direct patient care services, such as provider training, administrative meetings, and continuing medical education, in addition to clinical services.

However, the American Medical Association (AMA) [2] does not differentiate between these terms; it states that:

> the definition of telemedicine, as well as telehealth, has continued to evolve, and there is no consensus on the definition of either of the two terms.

According to state law in Oregon, USA [2]:

> the terms "telemedical services" or services delivered "telemedically" are also used and refer to telemedicine/telehealth.

The Telehealth Alliance of Oregon (TAO) suggests that [2]:

> you use definitions that are easiest for your organization to understand and implement internally. However, when working with other organizations, especially with regard to reimbursement, licensure or grants, it is important that you use the terms as they are defined by that organization.

After going through the opinions from these various reputed agencies, we can observe that some use these terms interchangeably. There is a thin line difference between these terms. The term *telemedicine* is related to providing clinical services, whereas the term *telehealth* covers all dimensions, including training and administration, as well as telemedicine [2]. In health informatics, the term *telehealth* encompasses telecare, telemedicine, and healthcare education, services and products. The term *telecare* is related to personal health tracking or self-care using mobile devices and alert systems based on ICT. Telemedicine has only a limited scope to provide healthcare to patients at distance, with remote communication between healthcare participants using digital transmission and fifth-generation cellular wireless networks (5G networks) [7, 8]. In a nutshell, the term *telemedicine* refers precisely to remote clinical services, while the term *telehealth* can refer to remote nonclinical services as well [8].

3.6 Examples and Uses of Telehealth and Telemedicine

- *Patient portals:* Instead of providing only an insecure means of communication with patients, a patient portal offers secure communication between patients and medical professionals, and it enables facilities such as prescription refills, clinical test results, a record of past visits and appointments, to name just a few [1].
- *Virtual appointments:* Another application can be virtual appointments with a doctor, which can occur through video conferencing, Web-based appointments, a call centre service, computer-driven decision-making and virtual visits [1].
- *Remote monitoring:* Remote monitoring enables a medical professional/doctor/healthcare professional to monitor a patient's health remotely using a Web-based or mobile app system. Remote monitoring also enables remote access to a patient's vital sign data via wearable devices or smart home monitoring devices [1].

- *Communication between doctors:* Using telehealth services, doctors can communicate with each other for consultations or discussions about patient care, research, patient referrals for better treatment, medical advice, and discussions about clinical test results [1].
- *Personal health records:* An electronic personal health record (PHR) app is accessible to patients 24/7 through Web-enabled devices, computers or smartphones. The PHR manages and stores data on the patient's history, medications, diagnostic and clinical test reports, and drug allergies, to name just a few aspects [1].

Thus, telemedicine is a medical tool that provides remote access and communication for patients and doctors [9].

3.7 Telemedicine Apps

Many mobile apps on smartphones (Android phones and iPhones) are designed to support better self-care and telemedicine. These mobile apps provide facilities to store personal health information, record data on patient vital signs, calculate and track food intake, schedule dosing reminders, record physical activity etc. [1]. Let us take a look at telemedicine apps that are popular among users, according to consumer reviews and user ratings (Table 3.1):

The major objectives of offering telemedicine apps are to provide 24/7 remote access and personal care, and to eliminate waiting times for patients, as well as for providers. The patient benefits include needs-based access to medical consultants, authorization to message a doctor, limited need for travel to a clinic, a lower cost of service, ease of use and accessibility. At the same time, these apps provide benefits for medical service providers, such as liberty to connect with remote doctors, access to home care and discharged patients, parallel patient consultation and treatment, access to electronic health records (EHRs) and other clinical systems, and fewer cancellations and missed appointments, to name just a few [5]. Telemedicine apps ensure provision of uninterrupted healthcare services and opportunities for users to rate them on the bases of services, quality and reliability [10].

3.8 Technology Requirements in Telemedicine

The technology requirements for telemedicine depend on the needs of the physician or the organization. The basic requirements for a telemedicine setup are [11]:

- *A secure broadband connection for remote connectivity:* An Internet connection with a connection speed of 50–100 megabits/second provides adequate video quality and adequate bandwidth and speed for data transfer.

Table 3.1 Telemedicine apps [10]

App	User ratings	Features
MDLIVE	iPhone rating: 4.7 stars Android rating: 4.7 stars	App for paediatric doctors providing behavioural health therapy services and psychiatry
Lemonaid—same-day online care	iPhone rating: 4.9 stars Android rating: 4.5 stars	Access to the Lemonaid pharmacy for diagnosis and treatment
LiveHealth Online Mobile	iPhone rating: 4.9 stars Android rating: 4.5 stars	Access to licensed therapists, lactation consultants, registered dietitians and other health professionals
PlushCare—video doctor visits	iPhone rating: 4.9 stars Android rating: 4.6 stars	Prescriptions, treatment, insurance information and connection to a doctor
Doctor on Demand	iPhone rating: 4.9 stars Android rating: 4.9 stars	Face-to-face consultation with a doctor, psychiatrist or psychologist whether the patient has insurance or not
Amwell—doctor visits 24/7	iPhone rating: 4.9 stars Android rating: 4.3 stars	Quality medical care and appointments on demand
Talkspace Therapy & Counseling	iPhone rating: 4.2 stars Android rating: 2.8 stars	A subscription service to improve mental health
Teladoc	iPhone rating: 4.8 stars Android rating: 4.6 stars	Connection to medical specialists virtually by video or audio chat, written prescriptions and expert medical advice
BCBSM Online Visits	iPhone rating: 4.9 stars Android rating: 4.7 stars	Physical and mental health services, and requests for care for children, too
Spruce—care messenger	iPhone rating: 4.9 stars Android rating: 4.8 stars	Dashboard for both providers and patients, protecting private medical information through HIPAA laws and allowing completion of essential health questionnaires and use of prewritten message templates

(continued)

Table 3.1 (continued)

App	User ratings	Features
Telehealth by SimplePractice	iPhone rating: 4.6 stars Android rating: 4.5 stars	Setup for virtual doctor's visits with a calendar system
DocsApp—consult a doctor	iPhone rating: 4.1 stars Android rating: 4.3 stars	Basic information about medical needs and connection with a medical provider quickly and virtually

HIPAA US Health Insurance Portability and Accountability Act of 1996

- *A video connection platform:* For video conferencing, this ranges from a basic setup on a home computer or an app-enabled smartphone to a secure video setup at a remote health centre, provided by a third-party vendor.
- *Technology support:* Virtual or in-person qualified computer and technical support are needed to provide uninterrupted Internet connectivity and to deal with technical and hardware problems.
- *Needs-based recording devices:* Typical video conferencing and third-party telemedicine systems provide provisions for recording and archiving of video. It is necessary to ensure adequate cloud storage and security.
- *Peripherals and video assist devices:* Peripheral devices are required to connect a few additional devices through universal serial bus (USB) connections, such as electronic stethoscopes, video otoscopes, dermascopes, telemedicine carts, and rolling or mobile devices. There is a need for computing devices with sufficient access, video equipment, and an uninterrupted power supply with adequate storage.

3.9 Features and Functionality of Telehealth Apps

To enable the complete features of telehealth services to be utilized with either a minimum viable product (MVP) or a fully featured telemedicine app, the following basic features are required in the app [5]:

- *An MVP feature set:* To provide basic features for remote and virtual care
- *Secure video calling:* For real-time, uninterrupted messaging and video conferencing
- *Peer-to-peer chat:* For exchange of multimedia content-rich messages
- *A back-end database and secure data warehouse:* For storing and authenticating patient data, health history data, laboratory test data and medical imaging data
- *Appointment scheduling:* To schedule appointments with medical consultants
- *An advanced feature set:* For additional features

- *Group chat and video calls:* Between doctors, between patients and doctors, and between doctors and pathologists/radiologists
- *Integration of the app with EHRs:* To collect patient history data for on-the-spot consultations
- *Virtual reality features:* For telepsychiatry during mental healthcare sessions
- *E-prescriptions:* For patients and doctors
- *A mobile payment gateway:* For payments to doctors
- *Integration with peripheral Internet of Things (IoT) devices:* To meet specific requirements for dentistry (teledentistry) or oncology
- *Integration with the Apple HealthKit and Google Fit:* For health and fitness–based apps
- *Built-in chatbots:* To provide additional help and answer frequently asked questions (FAQs)
- *A user interface for medical assistants and a dashboard:* For medical health workers to update health-related data/notes

The functionality of telemedicine relates to the processes to be followed to use the services. The purpose is to provide medical assistance to patients and remote connection with doctors. Traditionally, the service can be accessed via an online account or a tollfree phone number. The further process in a telemedicine service is shown in Fig. 3.1, demonstrating the overall functionality of using telemedicine [9, 12].

3.10 Setting Up a Telemedicine Program

To set up a telemedicine app, the designer and coder need to follow the steps listed in Fig. 3.2 [5, 13]:

3.10.1 Step 1: Select the Platform(s)

- Identify the platform(s), which will be iOS and/or Android for a mobile app, or the Web and/or a native platform for a desktop app.
- Select the target geography and the app functions/features.
- Select the appropriate platform on the basis of the predominant smartphone platform in the relevant geographical location. The predominant platform in the USA is iOS (55%); however, in most other countries, it is Android.
- Identify the appropriate application type (i.e. a mobile, Web-based or desktop-based application) on the basis of the target segment.
- Select a development tool (i.e. SaaS or a custom-based application using open-source or paid application programming interfaces (APIs)) on the basis of the development budget, development time and final cost to users.
- Analyse the cost-to-benefit ratio and the product–market fit.

Fig. 3.1 Functionality of telemedicine

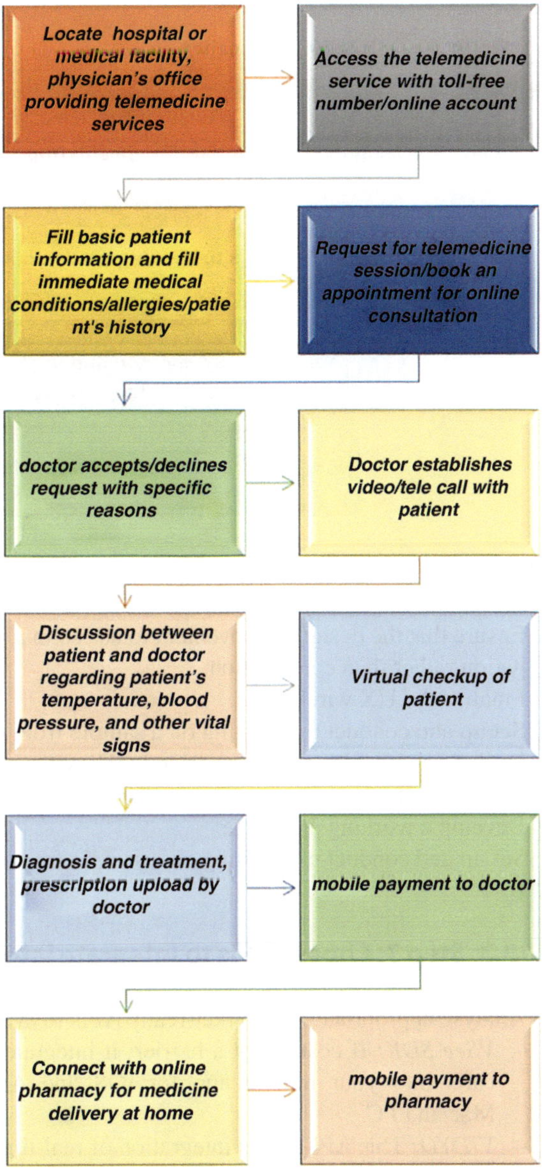

3.10.2 Step 2: Design an Appropriate App

- Select a user-friendly user interface and user experience (UI/UX) design.
- Plan the medical provider back-end and patient front-end UIs.
- Plan the content.

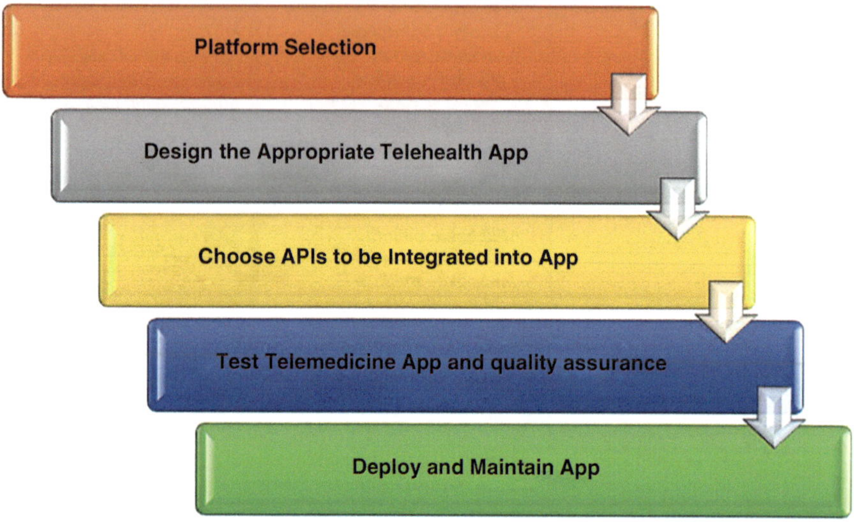

Fig. 3.2 Steps to set up a telemedicine program. *API* application programming interface

- Ensure that the design is convenient to use so that minimal time is spent on navigation rather than consultation.
- Finalize the UX wireframes.
- Set up and conduct user testing on a sample from the target segment.
- Design an interactive and user-friendly UI with suitable colours, theme, buttons, fonts and all other visual aspects of the app.
- Develop a working prototype.
- Set up and conduct user testing on a sample from the target segment.

3.10.3 Step 3: Choose APIs to Integrate into the App

- Analyse appropriate and market-ready APIs to avoid unnecessary delays:
  - *VSee SDK:* If cost is not a barrier; it integrates end-to-end encrypted video calls into your mobile app for iOS and Android, with native apps on Mac and PC.
  - *VIDYO:* This API allows integration of real-time communication capabilities into an app on Windows, Mac, Linux, iOS or Android; built-in text chat; and support for screen share and multiparty video calls.
  - *WebRTC:* Free and open-source platform; it is optimized to transmit audio, video and data; the supported browsers are Firefox, Opera, and Chrome on desktop and Android.
  - *OpenTok:* Cloud-based WebRTC platform; WebRTC is open source but OpenTok is not.
  - *Twilio:* APIs for SMS messaging, voice calls, text chat, email, fax and WhatsApp on all platforms.

- Select an appropriate API on the basis of the platform that is chosen and the features that are to be provided.

3.10.4 Step 4: Test the App and Perform Quality Assurance

- Ensure that the app works flawlessly.
- Execute peer code reviews through app developers.
- Carry out unit tests and frequent testing on various devices for quality assurance.
- Conduct quality assurance and regressing testing.
- Perform stress testing.

3.10.5 Step 5: Deploy and Maintain the App

- Deploy the app.
- Move the app to a live environment and into app stores.
- Market the app and provide customers with access to download it.
- Maintain and periodically update the app as per iOS and Android updates.

The cost of developing a telehealth app can vary from US$59,000 (using cross-platform mobile apps) to US$149,000 (for an advanced Web platform), depending the level of its complexity.

A study on patient satisfaction with telehealth found that patients considered convenience, efficiency, communication, privacy and comfort to be important parameters to consider when selecting a mobile app [14]. Hence, the setup and development of a telemedicine app should be centred around patient expectations.

3.11 Potentials and Limitations of Telehealth

The potentials of telehealth are as follows [1, 9, 12, 15–17]:

- It improves the quality of healthcare.
- It makes healthcare accessible to more people.
- It makes healthcare more efficient, better coordinated and available closer to home.
- It reduces the risks of contagion, hospitalization and death.
- It is helpful for patients in rural areas and those with mobility limitations.
- It is convenient for patients.
- A cash-only telemedicine service is less expensive than an urgent care clinic for patients. (Recently, the American Hospital Association reported on a telemedicine program that saved 11% in costs and more than tripled its investors' return on investment (ROI) [17].)
- Physicians do not lose money on cancellations or no-shows.

- Patients receive quick treatment, and physicians do not lose patients to quick-care retail clinics.
- It offers extended specialist and referring physician access.
- Patient engagement is increased.

The limitations of telehealth are as follows [1, 9, 12, 15–17]:

- Reduced care continuity may lead to gaps in care.
- Use of more than one telemedicine app may lead to overuse of medical care, inappropriate use of medications, or unnecessary or overlapping care.
- It does not really offer a complete alternative to a thorough physical examination and provides fewer in-person consultations.
- It is unsuitable for treating major injuries or illnesses.
- The security of personal health data can be compromised.
- Insurance services for telemedicine are limited, leading to greater out-of-pocket costs.
- It necessitates restructuring of information technology (IT) staff responsibilities and purchase of equipment, which are time consuming and costly.
- Policies and reimbursement rules can be problematic.

References

1. Mayo Clinic (2020) Telehealth: technology meets health care. https://www.mayoclinic.org/healthy-lifestyle/consumer-health/in-depth/telehealth/art-20044878#:~:text=Telehealth%20is%20the%20use%20of,or%20support%20health%20care%20services. Accessed on 13/5/2021
2. Telehealth Alliance of Oregon (2021) Telemedicine or telehealth—definitions. https://www.ortelehealth.org/content/telemedicine-or-telehealth-definitions. Accessed on 15/4/2021
3. American Hospital Association (2021) Fact sheet: telehealth. https://www.aha.org/factsheet/telehealth. Accessed on 15/4/2021
4. Global Telemedicine Market Growth, Trends | Industry Forecast 2021 to 2026 With COVID Impact - Mordor Intelligence. (n.d.). Mordor Intelligence. Retrieved May 3, 2021, from https://www.mordorintelligence.com/industry-reports/global-telemedicine-market-industry
5. Topflight Apps (2020) How to make a telehealth app: everything you need to know. https://topflightapps.com/ideas/how-to-create-a-telehealth-app/. Accessed on 12/3/2021
6. MedicAlert Advice (2021) Trends in telemedicine: 2021. https://www.medicalalertadvice.com/resources/telemedicine-trends/. Accessed on 12/3/2021
7. eVisit (2021) What is the difference between telemedicine, telecare and telehealth? https://evisit.com/resources/what-is-the-difference-between-telemedicine-telecare-and-telehealth/. Accessed 14/5/2021
8. American Academy of Family Physicians (2021) What's the difference between telemedicine and telehealth? https://www.aafp.org/news/media-center/kits/telemedicine-and-telehealth.html. Accessed on 14/5/2021
9. Berton R (2019) How to acquire access to telemedicine and telehealth services. Encore Telemedicine. https://encoretelemedicine.net/how-to-gain-access-to-telemedicine-services/. Accessed on 13/4/2021

10. Jewell T (2020) The best telemedicine apps of 2020. Healthline. https://www.healthline.com/health/best-telemedicine-iphone-android-apps. Accessed on 21/3/2021
11. Joshi M (2020) Telehealth Has Huge Potential, But Challenges Remain. Forbes. https://www.forbes.com/sites/forbesbusinessdevelopmentcouncil/2020/02/12/telehealth-has-huge-potential-but-challenges-remain/?sh=60872994191a. Accessed on 13/5/2021
12. eVisit (2021) How does telemedicine work? https://evisit.com/resources/how-does-telemedicine-work/. Accessed on 1/4/2021
13. Medscape (2021) Setting up a telemedicine program in your practice. https://www.medscape.com/courses/section/921364. Accessed on 11/5/2021
14. Powell RE, Henstenburg JM, Cooper G, Hollander JE, Rising KL (2017) Patient perceptions of telehealth primary care video visits. Ann Fam Med 15(3):225–229. https://doi.org/10.1370/afm.2095
15. Moneypenny M (2020) The enormous list of telehealth pros and cons. Etactics. https://etactics.com/blog/telehealth-pros-and-cons. Accessed on 1/4/2021
16. Harvard Health Publishing (2021) Telehealth: the advantages and disadvantages. https://www.health.harvard.edu/staying-healthy/telehealth-the-advantages-and-disadvantages. Accessed on 14/4/2021
17. eVisit (2021) 10 pros and cons of telemedicine. https://evisit.com/resources/10-pros-and-cons-of-telemedicine/. Accessed on 12/5/2021

4 Algorithms and Software for Smart Health

In Chapter 3, we discussed the technical requirements for telemedicine and provided a setup guide for it. In the same way, each smart health application (app) can be implemented or deployed using algorithms specific to the problem domain. The software apps used to implement a smart healthcare system will vary according to the technical requirements and budget.

This chapter covers various algorithms for developing smart healthcare apps and software for implementation. The chapter begins with software for telehealth. The subsequent sections cover different algorithms for healthcare, such as data science, artificial intelligence (AI), machine learning (ML), big data, the Internet of Things (IoT) and the cloud infrastructure. The chapter concludes by listing popular algorithms that are now used to transform healthcare.

4.1 Software for Telehealth

4.1.1 Security Regulations and Laws

Prior to planning and development of any telehealth apps, it is necessary to address the issues of security and risk, and to comply with the relevant regulations and laws [1]. These specify standardized practices for safe and controlled management of patient data. The following regulations and laws need to be followed in the development and operation of telehealth apps [1]:

- The Health Insurance Portability and Accountability Act of 1996 (HIPAA) regulations if the app will be used in the USA
- The General Data Protection Regulation (GDPR) if the app will be used in the European Union

S. Vyas, D. Bhargava, *Smart Health Systems*,
https://doi.org/10.1007/978-981-16-4201-2_4

- The Interstate Medical Licensure Compact (IMLC) if the app will be used in the USA
- The relevant regulations (including telemedicine regulations) in the country and/or state where the software will be used

4.1.2 Technology Stack for Telehealth App Development

Let us go through a technology stack commonly used to develop telehealth apps [1]:

4.1.2.1 WebRTC

WebRTC is a Web browser that provides application programming interfaces (APIs) to develop mobile apps enabling technology. It helps to create an appropriate user interface and user experience (UI/UX) for the apps. It provides a variety of features to be added into the app, such as text chat, secure voice conversations, screen sharing, live videos and store-and-forward data transfer.

4.1.2.2 Electronic Health and Medical Records Built on Rails and GraphQL

Rails and GraphQL provide support to build electronic health record (EHR) and electronic medical record (EMR) systems. These technologies provide storage, instant access, security, authentication and management of patients' information and histories.

4.1.2.3 Interactive Voice Response

Interactive voice response (IVR) is an automated telephony system technology that enables human–computer interface (HCI) through the IVR script and provides opportunities to implement voice and dual-tone multifrequency (DTMF) tones.

4.1.2.4 Cloud-Based Server Solutions

These are used to manage massive data storage requirements and to develop a communications platform over the cloud; cloud-based server solutions aid storage, security, exchange and management of medical/patient data over the cloud.

4.1.2.5 HealthKit Integration

HealthKit integrates health-monitoring and health-tracking platforms to develop telehealth apps. It provides an opportunity to use health-monitoring features and health data from smart wearable devices and smartphones. It also enables transfer of health data between patients and doctors.

Google Fit and Apple HealthKit are the most popular platforms of this type. Google has developed Google Fit for the Android operating system; it focuses more on medical/health data. For iOS, Apple HealthKit has been developed; its ecosystem consists of HealthKit (for fitness goals), CareKit (for self-care) and ResearchKit (for use by medical professionals).

4.1.3 Technologies Used in Telehealth Apps

In addition to the suggested technology stack for telehealth app development, let us go through the major technologies [1]:

According to an Accenture report, "AI-based medical and telehealth applications will reach around [US]$150 billion valuations in the healthcare industry by the end of 2026."

AI is one of the strongest technologies in telehealth. To provide effective communication between patients and doctors, AI-enabled chatbots can be implemented along with a voice search option. AI enables speech-to-text, frequently asked questions (FAQs), predictive search/suggestions and voice assistants to schedule appointments for patients, as well as for doctors.

AI and ML can also help to provide support for a disease diagnosis and recommendation system. In addition, AI-based telemedicine solutions can automate the basic workload of doctors in tasks such as notes management in EMRs, predictive diagnosis, and reminders, to name just a few.

Usually, augmented reality (AR) and virtual reality (VR) are used together to achieve various telehealth solutions. Using AR/VR, doctors can communicate with other medical teams and with doctors/surgeons in remote locations through video conferencing; can support each other in remote surgery, disease diagnosis and drug discovery; and can visualize their patients' data.

4.1.4 Guidelines for Building a Telehealth App

For successful development of any telehealth solution, the following guidelines should be followed:

1. Analyse the requirements and challenges to be addressed.
2. Identify the target segment and geographical specifications (if any).
3. Plan the major functionality and features of the telehealth solution as per the needs of the target audience.
4. Choose a multiplatform approach (e.g. using iOS, Android and a Web app) for health app development.
5. Select an appropriate tech stack to implement all desired features, keeping in view the software performance and server infrastructure.
6. Finalize appropriate UI/UX designs for a good functional user experience.
7. Have a vision for in-app integration with wearable devices, image-based consultation, chat integration etc.
8. Ensure that the app is secure.
9. Ensure that the app complies with the relevant legal regulations mentioned earlier.
10. Deploy secure authentication and data encryption in the app/software.

11. Conduct unit testing, integration testing, connectivity and compatibility checks, and quality assurance.
12. Collect user feedback on the app and maintain/update the app accordingly.

4.2 Softermii: Smart Healthcare App Development

The digital transformation in healthcare has brought about innovations in clinical practice, quality healthcare solutions and improved human lifespans. There is a need to ensure the security and adaptability of information and communications technology (ICT) to provide highly reliable health products, real-time clinical assistance, safe and secure environments, and high-quality healthcare.

The enormous growth in smart health initiatives and development of robust medical and wellness apps have empowered citizens to improve their lifespans and health, in addition to offering secure storage and organization of health data. One of the leading healthcare solution providers, Softermii, has successfully launched smart healthcare products for the medical industry [2].

Let us now take a brief look at a few solutions provided by Softermii for healthcare app development.

4.2.1 HIPAA Video

This is a Web-based doctor–patient video meeting platform, which provides a remote consultation feature for medical consultants and patients. Additionally, it also offers doctors a versatile dashboard for management or patient data.

4.2.2 Near Pharmacy

For the convenience of patients, the healthcare solution Near Pharmacy provides access to a nearby pharmacy. Patients can monitor a nearby pharmacy or their preferred drug stores, compare prices, define shopping preferences (online/offline), schedule deliveries and order/buy medicine offered through special deals. At the same time, Near Pharmacy provides pharmacists with the ability to target an audience with analytics.

4.2.3 PetRealTime

PetRealTime is a cloud-based solution that provides a communications platform for veterinarians and pet owners. To support veterinarians and pet owners, multipeer high-definition (HD) video streaming is provided for pet health consultations, progress follow-up, and appointments with veterinarians for physical visits.

4.2.4 Telehealth Apps and WebRTC

Telehealth solutions with WebRTC provide good-quality HD video for remote communication between practitioners and patients over the Web.

4.2.5 mHealth Apps

With the wide use of smartphones, user preferences for healthcare solutions have shifted towards mobile health apps. mHealth apps offer various facilities such as geolocation for healthcare practitioners and clinics, training and scheduling, customized hospital-related functions, doctors' feedback and referral services, medicine dosage and scheduling, and health monitoring, to name just a few.

4.2.6 IoT Firmware

IoT firmware includes IoT health devices and wearables to address fitness and health. Healthcare app development provides a highly iterative development environment to make use of IoT firmware integrated with any third-party components.

4.2.7 Medical Enterprise Apps

Medical enterprise apps provide a platform for medical institutions, hospitals and clinics to minimize the costs of services, optimize medical staff hours, and perform predictive functions for rapid emergency response.

4.2.8 Health Insurance Management

Health insurance management systems provide insurance and personal health data for patients, as well as for practitioners for the purpose of research.

4.2.9 Healthcare Data Security and Privacy Compliance

Healthcare data security provides security through encryption, safety, backup and recovery options for patient data to prevent unauthorized acquisition and potential loss due to system failure or malfunction. It prevents security breaches or hacking by privilege escalation.

A cross-dependent modular approach is employed to design a medical app with powerful logging abilities for administrators to see updates on the platform.

During mobile healthcare app development, the privacy and confidentiality of healthcare must be ensured, and, to protect and preserve all provider–patient interactions, the various necessary compliances must be ensured, such as compliance with HIPAA, the Health Information Technology for Economic and Clinical Health (HITECH) Act and the American Recovery and Reinvestment Act (ARRA) (in the USA); the GDPR (in the European Union); and other relevant state/country-specific laws, regulations and compliances.

4.2.10 Blockchain Ledger and EHRs

The blockchain ledger is supportable and acquiescent for EHR patient data. This technology complies with international health regulations and provides reliable platform storage and transfer of patient data.

4.3 Practice Management Solutions: Medical Practice Management Software

Practice management (PM) software is the most popular and inclusive type of software used to manage medical practices [3]. It provides a suite of services that fulfil all therapeutic practice requirements through a cloud-based system, including EHRs, EMRs, medical billing services, general administration and insurance checks, data and analytics for revenue cycles and workflows, a self-service patient portal and telemedicine software.

Let us explore PM suite services and medical PM software:

CareCloud Central is reputed cloud PM software, which offers a PM control centre to augment administrative and financial processes, a user-friendly interface and experience, EHRs and billing. The cost of the software is pocket friendly for developers and complies with global regulations and standards.

Eclipse PM software is the skilled veteran of PM, EHRs, and billing solutions, catering for single practices, multidisciplinary practices and multisite practices. This software platform is robust, cloud based, flexible and adaptable, and can be downloaded or executed from the cloud.

Greenway health is an inclusive and comprehensive cloud-based platform integrated with PM, EHRs, billing solutions, revenue cycle management (RCM), a clearinghouse, analytics and a speech-to-text feature.

Meditab is feature-rich adaptable practice software that includes EHRs and billing services. It also facilitates patient chart tracking, alerts and reminders; eligibility verification for insurance and insurance claim submissions; e-faxing; and analytical reports. Meditab was developed by doctors for doctors and provides support for hospitals, pharmacies and telemedicine.

AdvancedMD is a wider suite and integrated PM and medical billing software platform. It includes front-end office tasks, billing and payments, reporting and benchmarking tools, convenient scheduling and instant access to patient information. It also offers separate EHR software and a patient experience portal.

4.4 Problem-Specific Medical Algorithms Used in Smart Health

To provide better medical care, medical algorithms are integrated into the smart healthcare process and address specific healthcare challenges. Let us go through a few medical algorithms [2]:

4.4.1 Virtual Visit Algorithm for COVID-19 Patients

During the coronavirus disease 2019 (COVID-19) pandemic, virtual visits have become necessary to provide regular patient care and limit exposure to contagion. COVID-19 is considered a global emergency; across the globe, governments are encouraging use of telemedicine apps and solutions, and telehealth visits. Virtual visits include real-time audio/video-enabled telehealth visits, online e-visits, virtual check-ins, and telephone evaluation and management (E/M) visits. The virtual visit algorithm developed by James Dom Dera addresses the issues and procedures involved in all four types of virtual visits [4].

4.4.2 Telehealth Algorithm for Management of Dizzy Patients

A telehealth algorithm developed by Maaike Brons et al. addresses the issue of dizzy patients in a telemedicine setup. The algorithm, which is used for worsening heart failure, takes into account biometric measurements such as the body weight, blood pressure and heart rate [5].

4.4.3 QRS Detection Algorithm for Telehealth ECG Recordings

A QRS detection algorithm proposed by Khamis et al. provides a method for analysing clinical and telehealth electrocardiographic (ECG) data. It has been found to yield better results than the Pan–Tompkins (PT) and Gutiérrez-Rivas (GR) algorithms in the same domain area [6].

4.4.4 Other Medical Algorithms

These combat specific health issues such as diabetes, gastroesophageal reflux disease, chronic renal failure etc.:

- The Cambridge Diabetes Risk Score—a diabetes risk score for identifying patients in general practice at risk of type 2 diabetes mellitus [7]
- Alarm Symptoms for Patients with Gastroesophageal Reflux Disease [8]
- Occupational Risk Factors Associated with Development of Chronic Renal Failure [9]
- Risk Factors for Multidrug-Resistant Bacteria Causing an Exacerbation of Chronic Obstructive Pulmonary Disease (COPD) [10]
- The High Risk Alcohol Relapse (HAR) model [11]
- Use of artificial neural networks to identify patients with chronic low back pain conditions from patterns of sit-to-stand manoeuvres [12]

4.5 Algorithms Used to Transform Healthcare

4.5.1 Fourier Transform

The Fourier transform is a mathematical technique that can be used to support medical imaging, such as magnetic resonance imaging (MRI) and ultrasound imaging. It converts raw data into pictures and reduces the size of audio and image files into portable packages [13].

4.5.2 TCP/IP

TCP/IP is a common Internet standard for effective communication and medical data transfer in an agreed-upon format [13].

4.5.3 RSA Encryption Algorithm

The Rivest–Shamir–Adleman (RSA) encryption algorithm is used to encrypt electronic healthcare records and ensure their secure transmission [13].

4.5.4 MUMPS

The Massachusetts General Hospital Utility Multi-programming System (MUMPS) is a programming language for healthcare and supports clinical records management [13].

4.5.5 Probabilistic Data-Matching Algorithm

This is used by biologists in clinical research. It uses and ranks various bits of information in medical records and clinical data retrieved for research, and gives probability estimates for research hypotheses and genetic sequencing [13].

4.5.6 BLAST

The Basic Local Alignment Search Tool (BLAST) is a search algorithm for analysing gene and protein sequences. Biologists can use it to compare a sequence with others in a library or database of gene sequences for protein synthesis [13].

4.5.7 Neighbour-Joining Algorithm

This algorithm, paired with genetic sequencing, allows biologists to comprehend the evolutionary relationships among phylogenetic trees and drug development from natural substances. It also enables them to understand the adaptive evolution of bacteria, viruses and parasites, and behaviour such as infection of hosts, subversion of immune systems and resistance to treatment [13].

4.5.8 Medical Algorithms

These use evidence-based and data-driven approaches to help healthcare professionals understand medical errors and delivery of care, and to remove uncertainty from medical decision-making and improve its efficiency and accuracy [13].

4.5.9 Health Scores

These are scoring systems to determine the severity of patient illness in intensive care units (ICUs) and to help doctors monitor and predict multifactor patient diagnoses [13].

4.5.10 Big Data Analytics Tools and Techniques

Healthcare is a multidimensional system and is considered a big data repository comprising patient data, EHRs, medical imaging data, sociobehavioural data and environmental data. Big data in healthcare also include patient–provider data (EMRs), pharmacy prescription data and insurance records, genomics-driven experimental data and data acquired from smart wearables and IoT devices. Big data analytics stores sensing data, omics data, EHRs, public health records and clinical data in a data warehouse; performs data integration; performs analytics on these data (descriptive, diagnostic, predictive and prescriptive); and provides improved outcomes in the form of smarter and more cost-effective decisions. Hadoop, an open-source distributed app for big data, implements the MapReduce algorithm for processing and generating large data sets. At the same time, the Hadoop Distributed File System (HDFS) provides scalable, efficient and replica-based storage of medical data. An open-source alternative is Apache Spark, which provides scalability and built-in-fault-tolerance capability for big data analysis of medical data [14].

4.5.11 Quantum Algorithms

These can rapidity increase big data analysis and can reduce its information requirements and computational power requirements [14, 15].

4.5.12 Bioinformatics Tools for Medical Image Processing and Analysis

Bioinformatics software tools include VTK, ITK, DTI-TK, ITK-Snap, FSL, SPM, NiftyReg, NiftySeg, NifttSim, NiftRec, ANTS, GIMIAS, elastix, MIA, MITK, Camino, OsiriX and MRIcron, to name just a few. These algorithms can be used to analyse input images from sources of medical imaging (such as MRI, ultrasound, X-ray, functional MRI (fMRI), positron emission tomography (PET), computed tomography (CT), electroencephalography (EEG) and mammography), with graphical user interfaces and functions (generic, registration, segmentation, visualization, reconstruction, simulation and diffusion) [14, 16, 17].

4.5.13 Data Science Approaches

Data science algorithms for smart healthcare include principal component analysis, support vector machines (SVMs), linear/logistic regression, time series/sequence analysis, text mining, clustering, decision trees, visualization, K-nearest neighbours, the random forest algorithm, boosting, anomaly/deviation detection, ensemble methods, optimization and singular value decomposition, to name just a few [18].

4.5.14 AI and ML Approaches

Popular AI and ML algorithms for smart care include supervised and unsupervised algorithms such as SVMs to predict medication, protein classification, image segregation and text categorization; artificial neural networks (ANNs) for screening procedures such as Pap smears, mammograms and colonoscopy; deep learning models such as recurrent neural networks (RNNs) for pattern recognition in medical time–series data analysis and convolutional neural networks (CNNs) for multiclass classification problems and binary classification; discriminant analysis for EHR management systems and object classification; and naïve Bayes for medical data clarification and disease prediction [19].

References

1. Vaniukov S (2021) Telemedicine app development guide: benefits, features & cost. Softermii. https://www.softermii.com/blog/telemedicine-app-development-guide-benefits-technologies-features-to-watch-out. Accessed on 27/5/2021
2. Softermii (2021) Healthcare application development. https://www.softermii.com/solutions/healthcare. Accessed on 27/5/2021
3. Turner B (2021) Best medical practice management software of 2021. Techradar Pro. https://www.techradar.com/best/best-practice-management-software. Accessed on 30/5/2021
4. Dom Dera J (2020) A virtual visit algorithm: how to differentiate and code, telehealth visits, e-visits, and virtual check-ins. American Academy of Family Physicians. https://www.aafp.org/journals/fpm/blogs/inpractice/entry/telehealth_algorithm.html. Accessed on 28/5/2021
5. Chari DA, Wu MJ, Crowson MG, Kozin ED, Rauch SD (2020) Telemedicine algorithm for the management of dizzy patients. Otolaryngol Head Neck Surg 163(5):857–859. https://doi.org/10.1177/0194599820935859
6. Khamis H, Weiss R, Xie Y, Chang CW, Lovell NH, Redmond SJ (2016) QRS detection algorithm for telehealth electrocardiogram recordings. IEEE Trans Biomed Eng 63(7):1377–1388
7. Griffin SJ, Little PS, Hales CN, Kinmonth AL, Wareham NJ (2000) Diabetes risk score: towards earlier detection of type 2 diabetes in general practice. Diabetes Metab Res Rev 16(3):164–171
8. Min YW, Lim SW, Lee JH, Lee HL, Lee OY, Park JM, Choi M-G, Rhee P-L (2014) Prevalence of extraesophageal symptoms in patients with gastroesophageal reflux disease: a multicenter questionnaire-based study in Korea. J Neurogastroenterol Motil 20(1):87
9. Nuyts GD, D'Haese PC, Elseviers MM, de Broe ME, Van Vlem E, Thys J, De Leersnijder D (1995) New occupational risk factors for chronic renal failure. Lancet 346(8966):7–11
10. Chen G, Xu K, Sun F, Sun Y, Kong Z, Fang B (2020) Risk factors of multidrug-resistant bacteria in lower respiratory tract infections: a systematic review and meta-analysis. Can J Infect Dis Med Microbiol 2020:7268519
11. Yates WR, Booth BM, Reed DA, Brown K, Masterson BJ (1993) Descriptive and predictive validity of a high-risk alcoholism relapse model. J Stud Alcohol 54(6):645–651
12. Gioftsos G, Grieve DW (1996) The use of artificial neural networks to identify patients with chronic low-back pain conditions from patterns of sit-to-stand manoeuvres. Clin Biomech 11(5):275–280
13. Stewart K (2021) 10 algorithms that are changing health care. Algorithms for Innovation. https://uofuhealth.utah.edu/innovation/blog/2015/10/10AlgorithmsChangingHealthCare.php. Accessed on 15/5/2021
14. Dash S, Shakyawar SK, Sharma M, Kaushik S (2019) Big data in healthcare: management, analysis and future prospects. J Big Data 6:54. https://doi.org/10.1186/s40537-019-0217-0
15. Lloyd S, Garnerone S, Zanardi P (2016) Quantum algorithms for topological and geometric analysis of data. Nat Commun 7:10138
16. Schroeder W, Martin K, Lorensen B (2006) The visualization toolkit, 4th edn. Clifton Park, Kitware
17. Friston KJ, Ashburner JT, Kiebel SJ, Nichols TE, Penny WD (2006) Statistical parametric mapping: the analysis of functional brain images. Elsevier, London
18. Lytras MD, Chui KT, Visvizi A (2019) Data analytics in smart healthcare: the recent developments and beyond. Appl Sci 9(14):2812. https://doi.org/10.3390/app9142812
19. Rayan Z, Alfonse M, Salem ABM (2019) Machine learning approaches in smart health. Procedia Comput Sci 154:361–368

Scalable Smart Health Systems

5

In Chap. 4, we discussed various algorithms, tools and techniques for developing smart healthcare applications (apps). This chapter covers the concepts related to scalable smart healthcare systems, large-scale distributed computing in smart healthcare, and scalable and emerging smart healthcare systems.

5.1 Scalable and Emerging Smart Healthcare Systems

In this section, we review scalable and emerging smart healthcare systems such as IBM Watson, Open Mobile Health (Open mHealth), health decision support systems (HDSSs), the Stress Detection and Alleviation System (SoDA) and energy-efficient systems. Let us go through each of these systems in brief.

5.1.1 IBM Watson

According to an IBM Watson Redguide written by Rob High [1], IBM Watson is a cognitive system and can transform how organizations such as the healthcare industry align themselves as per the emerging requirements for scalability of smart healthcare systems. It provides capabilities for natural language processing (NLP) to understand the complexities of unstructured data, hypothesis generation and evaluation by applying advanced analytics to relevant evidence, and dynamic learning to improve learning on the basis of outcomes [1, 2].

Considering the massive volumes of medical data generated in real time in smart healthcare systems, the data can be unstructured and noisy, and can scale up. The big data generated through telemedicine or telehealth apps can be in different forms such as text forms (e.g. medical prescriptions), medical compliance documents for doctors (e.g. textbooks and guidelines), electronic medical records (EMRs) (e.g. text notes and images), health data (e.g. electronic health records (EHRs) and medical imaging data), telehealth software suites (e.g. user manuals, plans, guidelines

S. Vyas, D. Bhargava, *Smart Health Systems*,
https://doi.org/10.1007/978-981-16-4201-2_5

and proprietary data) and chatbots (e.g. frequently asked questions (FAQs)), to name just a few. IBM Watson provides an opportunity to store and manage such types of big data in the Watson corpus in the form of an extracted knowledge base. It also generates a distinct corpus per target domain [1].

Telemedicine apps provide an interactive platform for patients, as well as doctors, with smooth interaction. The deep NLP capabilities of IBM Watson use the Watson corpus to support typical chatbots, using question-and-answer-style inferences. The hypothesis generation capability of IBM Watson prepares a knowledge base from the history of patient–doctor conversations [1, 2]. The overall procedure is described below:

- When a patient poses a question, the Watson corpus captures all necessary features from the question, such as the name and age of the patient, any disease information and medical information.
- Further, it explores preprepared hypotheses generated by the corpus that are relevant to the patient's enquiry.
- It then matches the patient's answers with hundreds of hypotheses, using reasoning algorithms.
- It then selects the best match from the hypotheses that has the highest confidence score.

This approach does have limitations. It leads to high costs (as a large number of pages need to be acquired by the corpus), requires considerable processing power and has large memory requirements; yet, it is considered an appropriate approach in the healthcare domain.

The 'better-than-human content-reading capability' of Watson empowers smart healthcare to answer questions related to medical conditions or symptoms in the physical setting, as well as in the virtual clinic setting. The availability of enormous medical resources (such as healthcare/medical journals, patents, drug- and disease-related discoveries, clinical trial reports, EHRs, pathological and imaging data, and genomic data, as well as social content) allows Watson to scan and analyse content from a wide range of sources when preparing hypotheses [3].

This has led to the following major applications of Watson in healthcare.

5.1.1.1 Oncology

The major application of IBM Watson in oncology is called Watson for Oncology (WFO). It evaluates and ranks cancer treatment options by comparing a patient treatment with those described in relevant clinical trials/records. Its suggestion is based upon similar kinds of treatment prescribed in a similar category and intensity of other cancer cases. It gradually reduces the time and costs involved in extracting information from EHRs and medical journals [2]. Different researchers have stated that WFO is the preferred cognitive computing decision support system for cancers such as lung and colorectal cancer [4], breast cancer [5], colon cancer [6] and colorectal cancer [7], to name just a few.

5.1.1.2 Drug Discovery

IBM Watson for Drug Discovery (WDD) is a cognitive computing software approach for drug/pharmaceutical discovery [8]. In drug discovery, IBM Watson uses deep NLP-based extracts to cross-reference life science information on relevant drugs (chemical structures and action mechanisms) from sources identified as being effective for mitigation of specific disease. Watson further identifies original drug targets and identifies new uses for existing drugs. For example, Watson's deep NLP successfully identified 15 new drug candidates for treatment of a malaria parasite from a pool of drugs available from a pharmaceutical source [2, 3]. The hybrid approach to NLP in WDD incorporates a model-and-rule-based method and follows approaches such as entity recognition, entity resolution tasks and semantic relationship extraction [8].

5.1.1.3 Genomics

To enhance personalized treatment of patients with tumours, IBM Watson has the capability to extract new inferences and relationships between genes, proteins, drugs and diseases. It can rank and predict the most likely driver mutation and the type of DNA alteration in a patient's tumour [2].

WFO uses a clinical decision support system to provide prompt treatment recommendations for cancer patients. Similar research has been conducted by Liu et. al. in Chinese patients with lung cancer. It was observed that for the same patient, there was uniformity between the treatment recommendations for lung cancer made by WFO and those made by a multidisciplinary team (MDT) of practitioners [9].

An MDT is a multidisciplinary clinical decision–making team that provides patients with tailored treatment options. A retrospective research study found that there was some concordance between recommendations made by WFO and those made by an MDT [10].

5.1.2 Open mHealth

In a 2012 study by Localystics, it was stated that the Apple iPhone provided more than 13,000 health-related apps. An even greater number of such mobile healthcare apps are available for Android-based smartphones. Smart healthcare apps on smartphones and wearables facilitate storage of massive volumes of medical data related to EMRs and EHRs. In addition to the basic utility of these apps, they can also cater for management of chronic diseases. To address daily chronic disease prevention and assistance on the basis of these data, Open mHealth is a preferred choice [11].

Open mHealth provides a platform for patients with chronic conditions to record and track their vital physiological symptoms electronically. For instance, the WellDoc mobile diabetes management system can be used by patients with diabetes to store and track their blood glucose levels, and it also provides opportunities for their physicians to track their glucose levels to ensure that their treatment is adequate. This leads to reductions in clinical visits and emergency care use by these patients, with overall satisfaction for the patients, as well as for their physicians [12].

Open mHealth proposes use of open application programming interfaces (APIs) for fragmented mHealth apps deployed on mobile phones with a limited set of common communication protocols. This will also enable data transfer and use of application modules for multiple chronic diseases between multiple devices across multiple operating systems [11].

The standard data visualization tool InfoVis, developed in Open mHealth, offers special care for patients with posttraumatic stress disorder (PTSD). Such patients hardly ever pursue in-person consultations, because of stigma, logistical barriers, and overlooked symptoms. This tool enables direct visualization of self-reported PTSD, acute distress symptoms, checklist scores and blood glucose levels on the basis of data inputs from lower-level Lego-like reusable software modules: data processing units (DPUs) and data visualization units (DVUs) [13].

Dissimilar mHealth Apps usually do not interact or exchange data with each other, which makes complex behavioural interventions difficult. Open mHealth facilitates exchange of health information between mHealth apps. For behavioural interventions, an open-source extension to Open mHealth is proposed for Drishti (yogic gaze), using the sense–plan–act paradigm from robotics [14].

Sana is an open and customizable point-of-care platform for a mobile-based clinical information system. It connects workers and medical experts on a community health platform, allows doctors to encode new assessments, improves screening and diagnostics in resource-constrained settings, supports portable medical records, allows transfer of medical data from rural health workers to remote medical specialists for real-time decision support, and incorporates quality control and statistical analysis. Sana has been implemented for early detection of oral cancer in rural south India and for chronic diabetes management in Greece [15].

Open mHealth architecture is an engine for healthcare innovation in the management of chronic diseases (such as diabetes, asthma, and obesity) and for episodic care in a clinic/hospital-based setting. It supports medical discovery and evidence-based practice, and it provides opportunities to enhance disease prevention and management of chronic diseases [11].

5.1.3 Health Decision Support Systems

HDSSs have a multitier structure with a wearable medical sensor (WMS) tier and an ensemble of robust machine learning algorithms. They aid disease diagnosis and tracking by integrating WMS health data and a computer-based clinical decision support system (CDSS). They provide support for daily health monitoring, clinical checkups, thorough clinical examination, and postdiagnostic decision support through a pervasive health decision support (PHDS) system and a PHDS-assisted CDSS (CDSS+). PHDS uses WMS data for daily disease diagnosis, and CDSS+ handles clinical diagnosis.

An HDSS has four major tiers: tier 1 for daily health monitoring, tier 2 for immediate decision support for physicians, tier 3 for detailed diagnostic analysis and tier 4 for postdiagnostic treatment, prescription and lifestyle suggestions.

An HDSS uses two types of module: a disease diagnosis module for disease monitoring and a multiple disease diagnosis module to monitor various diseases in parallel.

An HDSS follows the World Health Organization's (WHO's) International Statistical Classification of Diseases and Related Health Problems (ICD) coding system for disease diagnosis module indexing [16].

5.1.4 SoDA Stress Detection and Alleviation System

SoDA, an automatic stress detection and alleviation system, is a user-friendly and user-transparent stress level coach. It uses WMSs to collect physiological signals and uses machine learning inferences (such as artefact removal, feature extraction, feature selection and principal component analysis) to provide stress level tracking and counselling [17].

SoDA regularly tracks physiological signals from patients to detect stress and guides the user whenever necessary. It assists patients suffering from major diseases such as cardiovascular diseases, sleep disorders and cancer. It provides high stress detection accuracy and efficient stress mitigation, using the following steps [17]:

- Extraction of physiological data from WMSs (using an individual/generalized operating model)
- Data cleansing of artefacts and extraction of informative features
- Input of feature values into a pretrained ML-based model
- Decision making under stressed/not stressed categories
- Use of a stress alleviation protocol
- Advice to the patient on stress-reducing therapies and analysis of extracted feature values from the collected physiological data
- Either termination of the stress alleviation protocol or continuation to the next stress-reducing therapy

5.1.5 Energy-Efficient Health Monitoring System

General-purpose health monitoring systems include implantable and wearable medical devices (IWMDs) and medical monitors powered by electrical outlets (e.g. on-site patient monitoring devices such as heart rate monitors, blood pressure monitors, oxygen saturation meters, accelerometers, electrocardiographs (ECGs) and electroencephalographs (EEGs)). IWMDs have constraints in terms of limited processing, storage and battery capacities. Developments in low-power wireless communications have enabled IWMDs to integrate with wireless body area networks (WBANs) to provide energy-efficient solutions with long-term continuous health monitoring.

Medical WBANs comprise biomedical sensors—low-sample-rate sensors (measuring the heart rate, blood pressure, oxygen saturation, temperature, blood sugar and accelerometry) and high-sample-rate sensors such as EEG and ECG sensors—connected with base stations/hubs such as mobile devices/smartphones, which aggregate medical data from biomedical sensors, using communications technology (radio and the ANT, ZigBee and Bluetooth Low Energy (BLE) protocols). To operate an energy-efficient health monitoring system, there is a need to reduce the energy consumption of each biomedical sensor. This can be done using sample aggregation, anomaly-driven transmission and sparse or compressive sampling (CS)–based computation and transmission. Of these three schemes, the CS-based scheme offers the greatest energy savings and low storage requirements [18].

5.2 Secure and Scalable Architecture Using Mist Computing

Mist computing is the combination of edge computing, fog computing and cloud computing. Mist computing is a low-power gateway and the extreme edge of a network. It makes use of micro-controllers and sensors to transfer data into fog computing nodes in order to use cloud computing services. Smart health provides telemonitoring by employing Internet-connected wearables; however, this may lead to long processing times and latency. To reduce latency and increase throughput, SoA-Mist (a three-tier secure framework–client layer, mist layer, fog layer and cloud layer) provides secure and scalable architecture for smart geospatial health data sets with use of mist devices (devices at the edge of the edge, such as cell phones, connected cars and smart home devices) [19].

5.3 Large-Scale Distributed Computing in Smart Healthcare

Smart health apps include remote health monitoring, wearable devices, activity recognition, mobile health and telehealth, and they generate massive volumes of big data to be managed through cloud computing. Such large-scale healthcare applications and architectures (or ubiquitous healthcare) need to provide high-performance solutions for smart healthcare. Large-scale distributed computing uses the Internet of things (IoT), big data analytics, fog computing, mobile health, large-scale medical data mining, machine learning and deep learning methods for processing multi-dimensional sensor data, smart homes, pervasive and context-aware computing, cloud computing, grid computing and resource allocation methods for BANs. For pervasive health monitoring and ambient-assisted living (AAL), smart healthcare systems employ high-performance computing (HPC) and large-scale distributed computing integrated with BANs to handle big data generated through smart wearables and heterogeneous devices [20].

5.4 Scalable Cognitive IoT–Based Smart City Network Architecture

The smart city includes smart buildings, smart homes, smart health, and smart industry. Cognitive IoT–based smart city network architecture provides scalability and flexibility, cognitive computing–based artificial intelligence (AI) solutions, human–machine interaction with personalized interactions and the capability to efficiently manage massive volumes of data (big data) in a smart city environment (such as healthcare, smart transportation, the retail industry and firefighting). The healthcare industry uses Welltok, a cognitive computing–based AI application; however, it does have limitations. Cognitive IoT–based smart city network architecture is implemented in the application layer of IoT for the purpose of creating intelligent environments to ensure data integrity, authenticity and confidentiality in smart buildings, smart homes, smart health, and smart industry [21].

Alhussein et al. [22] have proposed a cognitive IoT–cloud–based smart healthcare framework to deal with massive data volumes generated through medical devices/biomedical sensors (such as EEG sensors), with a deep learning–based EEG seizure detection method for smart city–based smart healthcare, using cognitive computing data [22]. Ahmed et. al. [23] have also highlighted the cognitive power of IBM Watson to transform global personalized medicine.

5.5 Cloud-Enabled WBANs for Pervasive Healthcare

We mentioned the WBAN concept in a previous section. Wan et al. [24] have proposed a scalable system architecture, BodyCloud (a cloud-enabled WBAN), for pervasive healthcare to manage spatial body sensor data. This architecture ensures scalability and flexibility of resources, sensor heterogeneity, and dynamic deployment and management of user and community applications [25].

For rapid prototyping of wireless body sensor network (WBSN) applications, the Signal Processing In-Node Environment (SPINE) domain-specific framework has been proposed by Bellifemine et al. [26]. The architecture of SPINE coordinates with the WBSN and sensors, evaluates different architectural choices and distributes signal processing and classification functions over the nodes of the network.

5.6 Blockchain-Based Distributed Architecture for a Scalable Smart City Network

Sharma et al. [27] have proposed DistArch-SCNet, a blockchain-based distributed architecture for a scalable smart city network. This architecture uses a light-fidelity (Li-Fi) communication technique to ensure scalability, efficiency, flexibility and availability in an existing smart city network.

5.7 Edge Computing for Scalable Smart Health

Edge computing capabilities and emerging wireless networking technologies provide real-time and cost-effective solutions for smart healthcare. The MEC-based architecture is a context-aware edge computing approach for efficient data delivery, multimodal data compression and edge-based feature extraction for event detection, ensuring high reliability and a rapid response [28, 29].

5.8 Structural Health Monitoring System for a Scalable Smart Sensor Network

Cho et al. [30] have deployed an autonomous structural health monitoring (SHM) system on a cable-stayed bridge (the Jindo Bridge in South Korea), using a dense array of a scalable smart wireless sensor network with 70 sensors and two base station computers. The aim is to ensure hardware durability, software reliability and low power consumption for efficient and autonomous monitoring of the bridge.

5.9 Fog Computing for Scalable Smart Healthcare

Fog computing is a distributed horizontal architecture—an alternative to the cloud—that exploits scalable computational/storage power and the edge-to-cloud network. Fog-based applications minimize round-trip delay overheads and implement a variety of low-latency services with minimal reliance on remote on-cloud resources for smart healthcare [2].

Okafor et al. [31] have proposed a fog computing network (FCN) for a scalable IoT data centre based on spine-leaf (SL) network topology. This solution addresses issues related to the Internet of Everything (IoE), such as huge traffic workloads, bandwidth, security and latency. There is a need to address the scalability requirements of smart healthcare applications in IoT data processing (such as assisted living systems, real-time analytics and smart embedded applications). This extended cloud IoT model optimizes bandwidth, allows global aggregation of edge devices, provides location awareness and low latency, and improves quality of service (QoS) performance. The fog distributed network includes real-time pooling, content caching at the edge, client-driven distributed broadcasts, client-to-client communication, cloudlets, smart over-the-top (SOTT) content management, radio network controllers, session management, ubiquitous crowd management, edge analytics, cognitive awareness, scalability and security [31]. Barik et al. [32] have also suggested the concept of Fog2Fog for health geographical information systems (GIS) to augment scalability in fog computing.

References

1. High R (2012) The era of cognitive systems: an inside look at IBM Watson and how it works. IBM, New York. http://www.redbooks.ibm.com/abstracts/redp4955.html?Open. Accessed on 25/5/2021
2. Yin H, Akmandor AO, Mosenia A, Jha NK (2018) Smart healthcare. Found Trends Electron Des Autom 12(4):401–466. https://doi.org/10.1561/1000000054
3. Chen Y, Argentinis JE, Weber G (2016) IBM Watson: how cognitive computing can be applied to big data challenges in life sciences research. Clin Ther 38(4):688–701. https://doi.org/10.1016/j.clinthera.2015.12.001
4. Somashekhar SP, Sepúlveda M-J, Norden AD, Rauthan A, Arun K, Patil P, Ethadka RY, Kumar RC (2017) Early experience with IBM Watson for Oncology (WFO) cognitive computing system for lung and colorectal cancer treatment. J Clin Oncol 35(15 Suppl):8527–8527. https://doi.org/10.1200/JCO.2017.35.15_suppl.8527
5. Somashekhar SP, Sepúlveda MJ, Puglielli S, Norden AD, Shortliffe EH, Kumar CR, Rauthan A, Kumar NA, Patil P, Rhee K, Ramya Y (2018) Watson for Oncology and breast cancer treatment recommendations: agreement with an expert multidisciplinary tumor board. Ann Oncol 29(2):418–423. https://doi.org/10.1093/annonc/mdx781
6. Lee WS, Ahn SM, Chung JW, Kim KO, Kwon KA, Kim Y, Sym S, Shin D, Park I, Lee U, Baek J-H (2018) Assessing concordance with Watson for Oncology, a cognitive computing decision support system for colon cancer treatment in Korea. JCO Clin Cancer Inform 2:1–8. https://doi.org/10.1200/CCI.17.00109
7. Kim EJ, Woo HS, Cho JH, Sym SJ, Baek J-H, Lee W-S, Kwon KA, Kim KO, Chung J-W, Park DK, Kim YJ (2019) Early experience with Watson for Oncology in Korean patients with colorectal cancer. PLoS One 14(3):e0213640. https://doi.org/10.1371/journal.pone.0213640
8. Martin RL, Martinez Iraola D, Louie E, Pierce D, Tagtow BA, Labrie JJ, Abrahamson PG (2018) Hybrid natural language processing for high-performance patent and literature mining in IBM Watson for Drug Discovery. IBM J Res Dev 62(6):8.: 1–8: 12. https://doi.org/10.1147/JRD.2018.2888975
9. Liu C, Liu X, Wu F, Xie M, Feng Y, Hu C (2018) Using artificial intelligence (Watson for Oncology) for treatment recommendations amongst Chinese patients with lung cancer: feasibility study. J Med Internet Res 20(9):e11087. https://doi.org/10.2196/11087
10. Tian Y, Liu X, Wang Z, Cao S, Liu Z, Ji Q, Li Z, Sun Y, Zhou X, Wang D, Zhou Y (2020) Concordance between Watson for Oncology and a multidisciplinary clinical decision-making team for gastric cancer and the prognostic implications: retrospective study. J Med Internet Res 22(2):e14122. https://doi.org/10.2196/14122
11. Estrin D, Sim I (2010) Open mHealth architecture: an engine for health care innovation. Science 330(6005):759–760. https://doi.org/10.1126/science.1196187
12. Quinn CC, Clough SS, Minor JM, Lender D, Okafor MC, Gruber-Baldini A (2008) WellDoc™ mobile diabetes management randomized controlled trial: change in clinical and behavioral outcomes and patient and physician satisfaction. Diabetes Technol Ther 10(3):160–168. https://doi.org/10.1089/dia.2008.0283

13. Chen C, Haddad D, Selsky J, Hoffman JE, Kravitz RL, Estrin DE, Sim I (2012) Making sense of mobile health data: an open architecture to improve individual- and population-level health. J Med Internet Res 14(4):e112. https://doi.org/10.2196/jmir.2152
14. Eapen BR, Archer N, Sartipi K, Yuan Y (2019) Drishti: a sense-plan-act extension to open mHealth framework using FHIR. In: Proceedings of the 2019 IEEE/ACM 1st international workshop on software engineering for healthcare (SHE), Montreal, 27–27 May 2019, pp 49–52. https://doi.org/10.1109/SEH.2019.00016
15. Behar J, Newton A, Dafoulas G, Celi LA, Chigurupati R, Naik S, Paik K (2012) Sana: democratizing access to quality healthcare using an open mhealth architecture. Int J Integr Care 12(4):e107. https://doi.org/10.5334/ijic.928
16. Yin H, Jha NK (2017) A health decision support system for disease diagnosis based on wearable medical sensors and machine learning ensembles. IEEE Trans Multi-Scale Comput Syst 3(4):228–241. https://doi.org/10.1109/TMSCS.2017.2710194
17. Akmandor AO, Jha NK (2017) Keep the stress away with SoDA: stress detection and alleviation system. IEEE Trans Multi-Scale Comput Syst 3(4):269–282. https://doi.org/10.1109/TMSCS.2017.2703613
18. Nia AM, Mozaffari-Kermani M, Sur-Kolay S, Raghunathan A, Jha NK (2015) Energy-efficient long-term continuous personal health monitoring. IEEE Trans Multi-Scale Comput Syst 1(2):85–98. https://doi.org/10.1109/TMSCS.2015.2494021
19. Barik RK, Dubey AC, Tripathi A, Pratik T, Sasane S, Lenka RK, Dubey H, Mankodiya K, Kumar V (2018) Mist data: leveraging mist computing for secure and scalable architecture for smart and connected health. Procedia Comput Sci 125:647–653. https://doi.org/10.1016/j.procs.2017.12.083
20. Khan SU, Zomaya AY, Abbas A (eds) (2017) Handbook of large-scale distributed computing in smart healthcare. Springer, New York. https://doi.org/10.1007/978-3-319-58280-1
21. Park J-H, Salim MM, Jo JH, Sicato JC, Rathore S, Park JH (2019) CIoT-Net: a scalable cognitive IoT based smart city network architecture. Hum-centric Comput Inf Sci 9(1):190. https://doi.org/10.1186/s13673-019-0190-9
22. Muhammad G, Hossain MS, Amin SU (2018) Cognitive IoT-cloud integration for smart healthcare: case study for epileptic seizure detection and monitoring. Mob Netw Appl 23(6):1624–1635. https://doi.org/10.1007/s11036-018-1113-0
23. Ahmed MN, Toor AS, O'Neil K, Friedland D (2017) Cognitive computing and the future of health care cognitive computing and the future of healthcare: the cognitive power of IBM Watson has the potential to transform global personalized medicine. IEEE Pulse 8(3):4–9. https://doi.org/10.1109/MPUL.2017.2678098
24. Wan J, Zou C, Ullah S, Lai C-F, Zhou M, Wang X (2013) Cloud-enabled wireless body area networks for pervasive healthcare. IEEE Netw 27(5):56–61. https://doi.org/10.1109/MNET.2013.6616116
25. Fortino G, Pathan M, Di Fatta G (2012) Body cloud: integration of cloud computing and body sensor networks. In: Proceedings of the 4th IEEE international conference on cloud computing technology and science, Taipei, 3–6 Dec 2012; pp 851–856. https://doi.org/10.1109/CloudCom.2012.6427537
26. Bellifemine F, Fortino G, Giannantonio R, Gravina R, Guerrieri A, Sgroi M (2011) SPINE: a domain-specific framework for rapid prototyping of WBSN applications. Softw - Pract Exp 41(3):237–265. https://doi.org/10.1002/spe.998
27. Sharma PK, Rathore S, Park JH (2018) Dist Arch-SCNet: blockchain-based distributed architecture with Li-Fi communication for a scalable smart city network. IEEE Consum Electron Mag 7(4):55–64. https://doi.org/10.1109/MCE.2018.2816745
28. Abdellatif AA, Mohamed A, Chiasserini CF, Tlili M, Erbad A (2019) Edge computing for smart health: context-aware approaches, opportunities, and challenges. IEEE Netw 33(3):196–203. https://doi.org/10.1109/MNET.2019.1800083
29. Akmandor AO, Jha NK (2018) Smart health care: an edge-side computing perspective. IEEE Consum Electron Mag 7(1):29–37. https://doi.org/10.1109/MCE.2017.2746096

30. Cho S, Jang SA, Jo H, Mechitov K, Rice JA, Jung H-J, Yun C-B, Spencer BF Jr, Nagayama T, Seo J (2010) Structural health monitoring system of a cable-stayed bridge using a dense array of scalable smart sensor network. In: Proceedings of SPIE smart structures and materials + nondestructive evaluation and health monitoring, San Diego, 7–11 Mar 2010. https://doi.org/10.1117/12.852272
31. Okafor KC, Achumba IE, Chukwudebe GA, Ononiwu GC (2017) Leveraging fog computing for scalable IoT datacenter using spine-leaf network topology. Int J Electr Comput Eng 2017:2363240. https://doi.org/10.1155/2017/2363240
32. Barik R, Dubey H, Sasane S, Misra C, Constant N, Mankodiya K (2017) Fog2Fog: augmenting scalability in fog computing for health GIS systems. In: Proceedings of the 2017 IEEE/ACM international conference on connected health: applications, systems and engineering technologies (CHASE), Philadelphia, 17–19 Jul 2017, pp 241–242. https://doi.org/10.1109/CHASE.2017.83

Devices, Systems and Infrastructures for Smart Health

6

Health is the most important aspect of human life, and smart health can be considered a current revolution in health. There is an increasing need for smart technologies to provide disease diagnosis and healthcare treatment, using the most efficient and reliable sources of information, and with rapid increases in technology, smart health systems are being upgraded. Nowadays, a detailed report on the human body can be obtained by collecting data with particular Internet of Things (IoT) devices, and many important tests on the human body can be done easily by a few sensors in a very short period of time. Reports can also be analysed remotely by experts when no appropriate specialist is available locally. Smart healthcare systems are also cost effective for provision of medical services. Nowadays, IoT devices and sensor systems are used widely in smart healthcare systems [1]. A radical upgrade of the traditional healthcare system is the need of the hour, and that gap can be filled only by implementation of smart health services. These services involve smart infrastructure to build smart systems with smart IoT devices to track the health of patients. Such devices help to provide efficient, fast and precise disease diagnoses and determine what treatment should be used. Sensor-based devices create a customized system for a patient or user by formulating the results obtained from the data sets provided by these smart devices. This whole system creates a responsive framework and a smart infrastructure for smart health. This infrastructure is based purely on the feedback given by the sensors in the form of data; the data are then analysed by algorithms, and suitable actions can then be taken as a result of these sequences. Moreover, IoT devices used in smart health can provide full 24/7 observations of the patient, tracking and measuring progress in terms of data sets, which can then be further utilized by doctors to provide better treatment for the patients.

This chapter analyses the needs of smart healthcare infrastructures and smart devices that help to transform healthcare systems into smart ones. Smart healthcare devices can be capable of multidisciplinary use, and single devices can be used and reused, with customizable programming algorithms being installed to perform different operations.

S. Vyas, D. Bhargava, *Smart Health Systems*,
https://doi.org/10.1007/978-981-16-4201-2_6

The basic infrastructure and classification of smart health system operations are as follows (Fig. 6.1):

- Sensor data are acquired by the system.
- The data are cleaned and processed.
- The data are normalized.
- Informative features selection.
- The selected features are analysed to assess whether a health alert should be triggered.
- If an alert is triggered, either the necessary tasks are performed or users are guided appropriately [2].

The main purpose of smart IoT devices in the field of healthcare is to provide improved medical amenities for patients, medical staff and medical care units [3]. Smart devices can easily generate alerts about users' or patients' critical conditions and send them to their doctors in real time over the Internet [4]. Predictions made by smart healthcare devices using data mining are a very powerful technology, which uses existing databases to analyse the results according to defined parameters [5]. This technology supports doctors in identifying diseases with the help of previously saved data from past treatments. Smart healthcare can be used for early detection and prevention of serious complications or life-threatening disease.

6.1 Smart Health Infrastructures

In the present technological revolution, there is a great need to change the healthcare industry through automation, which is perhaps as urgent as it is difficult. The term *smart health* refers to information technology (IT) infrastructures and technologies that are helping to improve the activities of the healthcare industry and making its processes more automated and more specialized [6]. Smart healthcare infrastructures (see Fig. 6.2) comprise optimized and automated processes utilizing standard communication and technological environments [7]. The main purpose of

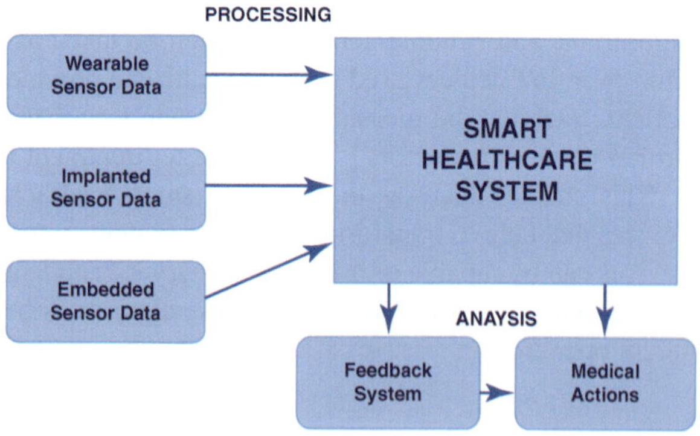

Fig. 6.1 Smart healthcare system

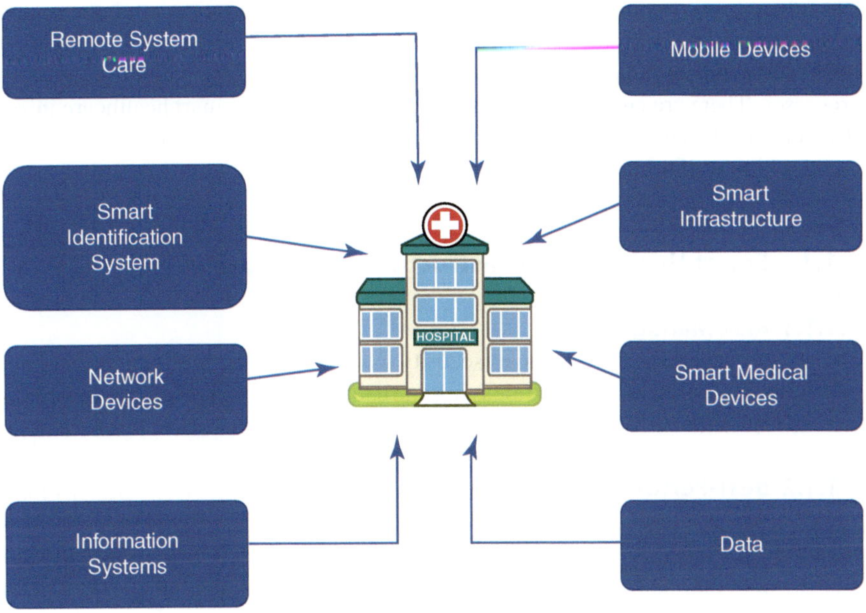

Fig. 6.2 Smart infrastructure of a healthcare system

every smart health infrastructure is to upgrade conventional procedures to more advanced ones. Remarkable results have been observed when such advancements have been made in the healthcare sector. The healthcare infrastructure is being totally transformed by use of connected and sensor-based devices. However, these advancements entail some challenges and risks such as loss of patients' health information and personal data, system failures and natural disasters. The incidence of malicious attacks has also increased exponentially because of the connection of these devices [8]. As everything around the globe is digitizing, so are the services and experiences of patients at healthcare centres. Patients are dealing with sensor-based smart devices, remote access devices and smart gadgets with great ease. Healthcare systems are utilizing smart devices, electronic health records (EHRs) and tablets for recording, monitoring and storing patient records. These smart techniques and devices also provide better-quality care and tracking of patients' health and other relevant information. As per the needs of society, smart healthcare infrastructures are becoming essential.

There are many threats associated with healthcare systems. Threats such as human error, malicious actions, system failures and third-party technical errors pose risks and vulnerabilities in a healthcare system. A well-secured system requires efficient security measures and compliance standards, with proper training of staff and appropriate awareness. Healthcare systems also need to follow guidelines and well-framed security procedures such as encryption techniques, intrusion detection, system monitoring and configuration management. Information systems in smart healthcare need to incorporate security procedures and secure devices [9]. It is said that a healthcare system is smart when it makes use of optimized and automated processes created using an IoT-based information and communications technology (ICT) environment of connected devices for improving existing patient-monitoring processes. There are enormous cybersecurity challenges in a smart healthcare infrastructure. To deal with all of these challenges, there is a specific framework according to which configuration can be done.

6.1.1 Smart Healthcare Infrastructure Challenges

6.1.1.1 Risk Management

This is a six-layer approach to smart security that offers the capability for detecting, delaying, defending against and denying intrusion and security failures in healthcare infrastructures.

6.1.1.2 Best-Performance Networks

For a better performing healthcare system, a highly efficient networking system is essential. With this, it becomes easy to have versatile connections in the physical layer of networks to support multiple applications with increases in bandwidth and much less network downtime.

6.1.1.3 Power Optimization

When critical power is being considered in a healthcare environment, multiple factors such as facilities, backup, and conditioned, efficient and monitored power must be considered. Development of a critical power chain that starts in the grid and flows through the healthcare equipment and devices will make sure those considerations are addressed.

6.1.1.4 Communication Efficiency

Communication is a very important factor in consideration of patient care. Improving responsiveness, providing seamless wireless availability and reducing noise pollution require targeted healthcare engagement, where new technologies can simplify the flow of information between healthcare staff, patients and administrators.

6.1.1.5 IoMT Enablement

Internet of Medical Things (IoMT) enablement is helpful for making real-time modifications and analysing the healthcare environment to improve efficiency and productivity.

Advances in healthcare systems play an important role in transforming conventional cities into smart cities. ICT research and advancements have transformed healthcare services into smart ones with better quality and efficiency. Applications related to smart healthcare systems plays a vital role in improving the quality of healthcare processes and reducing the complexities of healthcare services [10]. Smart devices are an important part of smart healthcare systems, as they can assist monitoring of health and provide necessary medications for patients. Data provided by smart devices are accessed and analysed by healthcare workers, professionals and researchers for more efficient diagnosis and treatment through interaction with smart healthcare technologies. Digital records provided by smart devices identifies details related to personal medication and treatment procedures, of patients and staff, which saves both cost and time. These records also provide the opportunity for preventive procedures via real-time data collection [11].

6.2 Smart Healthcare Structures

A smart healthcare system is purely a system of interconnected IoT devices. Nowadays, the Internet plays a crucial role in our lives. It has transformed the life-styles of people, and it serves almost every sector of human life. The next major innovative move is IoT and its devices [12], which connect small objects to the Internet. The communication between these devices is fast, reliable and secure. Depending on the different applications that are used, there are many devices available for a smart healthcare system. Many of them are wearable, implanted and embedded devices [2].

A smart healthcare monitoring system consists of a collection of various subsystems (see Fig. 6.3), which are described below.

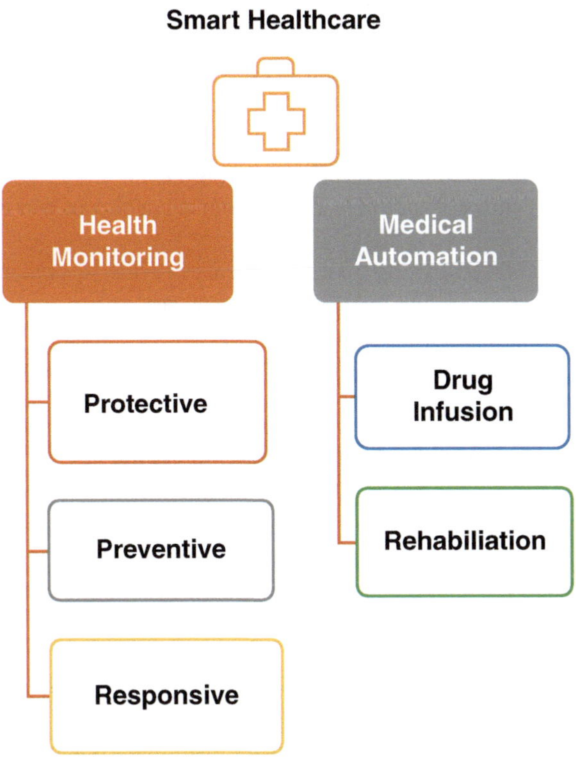

Fig. 6.3 Classification of a smart healthcare system

6.2.1 Protective Systems

These types of system are used for tracking patients' health and for regular checks. They generate health-related alert notifications to their users. Such protective systems are categorized into two main parts:

- *A pre-incident system:* This system gives an indication regarding the health of a person to provide information on incidents or situations that may lead to critical problems.
- *A post-operative system:* This system makes use of health indicators to detect infections or complications after procedures or surgery.

6.2.2 Preventive Systems

These are smart healthcare systems for detecting unhealthy conditions in patients and also provide practical approaches to deal with such situations. These systems can take preventive measures before a medical situation arises [2]. Systems such as fitness tracking devices, stress management devices and other monitoring devices fall into this category. Preventive systems are used to prevent disease through tracking and guidance regarding the appropriate measures to be taken in order to maintain a healthy lifestyle.

6.2.3 Responsive Systems

These are smart systems that help to diagnose disease early by tracking a patient's health continuously and generating health alerts. Disease can be identified from very minor symptoms. These systems are also of two types:

- *Emergency care:* These systems provide responsiveness by being activated in scenarios that warrant emergency care.
- *Regular care:* These systems provide responsiveness in terms of regular care of the user by continuously tracking activities and incidents.

6.2.4 Medical Automation Systems

Such smart healthcare systems are sensor-based wearables and ingestibles for providing medical support for the user. They help by providing alerts regarding medication and health consultations and by keeping a continuous track of the user's health record. Such systems are categorized into two parts:

- *Drug infusion systems:* These systems help to inject an exact amount of medicine into the patient's body. This is done with the help of digitally connected systems—for example, to deliver insulin to a diabetic patient or to deliver morphine for pain relief.

- *Rehabilitation systems:* These systems help to improve the physical abilities of the user after a serious stroke, traumatic injury or other serious incidents. These systems support the user by providing objective acknowledgements [2].

6.3 Smart Healthcare Devices

IoT-based smart healthcare systems help to keep track of patients' health on a 24/7 basis. IoT sensors have become a very reliable source of information in the healthcare field; moreover, these devices do not need any secondary verification of their reports to the user [14]. As a result of advancements in very large-scale integration (VLSI) technology, sensors are becoming smaller and can be used as wearables.

The benefits of smart healthcare devices are as follows [13]:

- Instantaneous reporting and treatment
- End-to-end connection
- Data analysis and collection
- Alert generation and monitoring
- Remote medical support

The challenges associated with smart healthcare devices are as follows [13]:

- Security and confidentiality
- Integration of devices, procedures and technology
- Data accuracy and reliability
- Pricing and resources

Smart healthcare devices consist of three major device categories:

- Sensor-based smart healthcare monitoring devices
- Smartphone-based smart healthcare monitoring devices
- Microcontroller-based smart healthcare monitoring devices

6.3.1 Sensor-Based Smart Healthcare Devices

Sensor-based smart healthcare devices collect data related to the patient's health via electronic data signals and then generate alerts. The most widely used sensors are electrocardiography (ECG) sensors, heat sensors and pulse rate sensors. Some sensors that are very important and are used for specific purposes are radiofrequency identification (RFID)–based sensors, humidity sensors, biomechanical sensors, glucose meter sensors, body posture sensors and respiration sensors [15].

Small sensors can be placed all over the body and connected to a wireless body area network (WBAN) to help the relevant people or doctors to make extra observations of the patient. All of the sensors are connected to the Internet and work as per their responsibilities.

6.3.2 Smartphone-Based Smart Healthcare Devices

Smartphones have proved to be a most valuable resource worldwide. There are a significant number of features in a smartphone that can serve the smart healthcare system in many ways. Smartphones have different types of sensors embedded as features, which then can be used to take input from the user. These sensors include wireless and Bluetooth sensors, Global Positioning System (GPS) trackers and biometric sensors. The most important aspect of using a smartphone is that it can also store data, so when data on the user are collected with the help of sensor applications, they can be stored locally and transmitted via the Internet [16]. Smartphones cannot generate data as accurate as those generated by wearable devices or body-embedded sensors, but they can give a rough idea of the status or condition of the user. Smartphones are becoming a very crucial part of human lives, and easy-to-use configurations can help smart healthcare systems collect data via use of smartphones.

6.3.3 Microcontroller-Based Smart Healthcare Devices

Microcontrollers have proved to be very useful and important devices when it comes to healthcare monitoring structures. Microcontrollers work comparatively fast and can process huge data sets in a very short time. These controllers are used as an interface for sensors, as they are very small and thus can effectively produce mobile data. Many microcontroller-based frameworks, such as the Raspberry Pi, are now commonly used in healthcare systems. In contrast, Arduino Uno is not that appropriate for managing more than one sensor at a time but does allow inputs to be obtained and then formulated according to the requirements. Microcontrollers can also be used to troubleshoot existing smart healthcare devices in order to improve the accuracy of the devices. Smart healthcare systems can be created with the help of different microcontrollers in any environment. There have been a number of competitions and hardware hackathons in which healthcare students have used microcontrollers. However, it is very difficult to embed every required element of the system into a single device so that microcontrollers can be independent and highly mobile, which would be an advantage for such devices.

6.3.4 IoT/IoMT/Sensor-Based Healthcare Devices

These include the following [14]:

- Remote patient-monitoring devices
- Smart data transmission tools
- Sensor-based air, water and food quality–testing devices
- Drug efficiency trackers
- Smart medical data–capturing devices
- Glucose-monitoring and heart rate–monitoring devices

- Biometric care scanners
- Sleep-monitoring and safety devices

Smart healthcare has changed the face of the healthcare industry by providing smart and efficient facilities to monitor and manage patients' health information. Sensor-based and embedded smart healthcare systems provide healthcare personnel with more intensive and more accurate data, which help them to track and medicate patients in an improved manner. These sensor-based devices still require further refinement for better compatibility with the edge-side requirements of healthcare systems. These requirements can be related to security and privacy, smart planning, decision making, and tracking and monitoring. To fulfil the needs of smart healthcare systems, smart tools, techniques and models need to be designed that overcome various challenges such as cost, operability, accuracy, scalability and reliability. These smart healthcare systems need to be more personalized to record and analyse more intensive and more accurate data (related to the patient's age, heart rate, pulse, blood sugar level etc.) because use of inaccurate data may lead to adverse events. To achieve accuracy and efficiency in use of healthcare data, use of smart technologies (such as IoT, big data and artificial intelligence (AI) frameworks, models and devices) is now causing a revolution in the healthcare industry. IoT has the potential to excel in smart health with the help of smart infrastructure, systems and devices together. The main reason to use smart health with IoT is to enhance the mobility of the devices and the availability of resources. This will benefit everybody, particularly people living in remote locations far from medical services [17]. Smart healthcare systems are advantageous for patients and also for society, as implementation of these systems will bring efficiency, robustness and also reductions in the costs and time involved in healthcare delivery.

References

1. Rahaman A, Islam MM, Islam MR, Sadi MS, Nooruddin S (2019) Developing IoT based smart health monitoring systems: a review. Revue d'Intelligence Artificielle 33(6):435–440. https://doi.org/10.18280/ria.330605
2. Akmandor AO, Jha NK (2017) Smart health care: an edge-side computing perspective. IEEE Consum Electron Mag 7(1):29–37. https://doi.org/10.1109/MCE.2017.2746096
3. Banka S, Madan I, Saranya SS (2018) Smart healthcare monitoring using IoT. Int J Appl Eng Res 13(15):11984–11989
4. Pandey H, Prabha S (2020) Smart health monitoring system using IoT and machine learning techniques. In: Proceedings of the 2020 sixth international conference on bio signals, images, and instrumentation (ICBSII), Chennai, 27–28 Feb 2020, pp. 1–4. https://doi.org/10.1109/ICBSII49132.2020.9167660
5. Mohapatra S, Patra PK, Mohanty S, Pati B (2018) Smart health care system using data mining. In: Proceedings of the 2018 international conference on information technology (ICIT), Bhubaneswar, 19–21 Dec 2018, pp 44–49. https://doi.org/10.1109/ICIT.2018.00021
6. Incepta (2020) Smart hospitals—an insight into healthcare infrastructure automation. https://www2.inceptasolutions.com/2020/03/12/smart-hospitals-an-insight-into-healthcare-infrastructure-automation/. Accessed on 20/03/2020
7. European (Union Agency for Network and Information Security (ENISA) (2016)

8. AET (2017) Smart hospitals: security and resilience for smart health service and infrastructures. https://www.aeteurope.com/news/smart-hospitals-security/. Accessed on 10/03/2020
9. European Union Agency for Cybersecurity (2016) Cyber security and resilience for smart hospitals. https://www.enisa.europa.eu/publications/cyber-security-and-resilience-for-smart-hospitals. Accessed on 12/03/2020
10. Sanghavi J (2020) Review of smart healthcare systems and applications for smart cities. In: Kumar A, Mozar S (eds) ICCCE 2019: proceedings of the 2nd international conference on communications and cyber physical engineering. Springer, Singapore, pp 325–331. https://doi.org/10.1007/978-981-13-8715-9_39
11. Choudhary M (2019) Smart healthcare for a healthy smart city. Geospatial World. https://www.geospatialworld.net/blogs/smart-healthcare-for-a-healthy-smart-city/. Accessed on 10/03/2020
12. Budida DAM, Mangrulkar RS (2017) Design and implementation of smart healthcare system using IoT. In: Proceedings of the 2017 international conference on innovations in information, embedded and communication systems (ICIIECS), Coimbatore, 17–18 Mar 2017, pp 1–7. https://doi.org/10.1109/ICIIECS.2017.8275903
13. Peerbits (2021) Internet of things in healthcare: applications, benefits, and challenges. https://www.peerbits.com/blog/internet-of-things-healthcare-applications-benefits-and-challenges.html. Accessed on 20/03/2021
14. Pradhan B, Bhattacharyya S, Pal K (2021) IoT-based applications in healthcare devices. J Healthc Eng 2021:6632599. https://doi.org/10.1155/2021/6632599
15. GlobalData (2019) Wearable technology in healthcare—thematic research. https://store.globaldata.com/report/gdhcht026%2D%2Dwearable-technology-in-healthcare-thematic-research/#product-1340945. Accessed on 10/03/2020
16. Pasha M, Shah SMW (2018) Framework for E-health systems in IoT-based environments. Wirel Commun Mob Comput 2018:6183732. https://doi.org/10.1155/2018/6183732
17. Baker SB, Xiang W, Atkinson I (2017) Internet of things for smart healthcare: technologies, challenges, and opportunities. IEEE Access 5:26521–26544. https://doi.org/10.1109/ACCESS.2017.2775180

Cyber-physical Systems for Healthcare

7

Cyber-physical systems (CPSs) for healthcare are also known as medical cyber-physical systems (MCPSs) and can be thought of as mechanisms that integrate physical and computational methods. They are deployed via monitoring of computer-based algorithms fused with the Internet. They also serve as a bridge between the virtual and physical worlds [1]. These new-generation systems are combined engineered systems consisting of electrical technology, communications technology, information technology and control systems. CPSs play important roles in the area of healthcare and information systems. There are numerous applications utilizing CPS, such as healthcare, traffic management systems, information systems and transportation systems. CPSs have revolutionized many areas such as healthcare monitoring, responses to emergency situations and delivery systems. CPSs integrate physical and logical areas by putting digitized, physical and human elements together in unified processes. CPSs includes technologies such as the Internet of Things (IoT), smart cities, smart healthcare and, indeed, 'smart' anything (buildings, vehicles etc.)

It has recently been observed that smart healthcare systems integrated with CPSs can help and transform the healthcare sector completely. This has proved to be beneficial in providing more convenient facilities and conditions for healthcare systems. The Internet has transformed the new technological generation of systems for healthcare by integrating control and computational proficiencies. CPSs are used in hospitals to produce results quickly and efficiently, improving the quality of the healthcare that is provided. At present, the CPS concept is still evolving and presents certain challenges, and further research on CPSs is needed in the area of healthcare. Use of wireless sensor networks plays an important part in CPSs because they enable robust sensor capability. CPSs are smart, dynamic and adaptive, which makes this technology distinctive and multivalued.

This chapter discusses the needs, technological aspects, architecture, applications and benefits of CPSs, along with the challenges related to these emerging technologies and the future of these systems in healthcare.

S. Vyas, D. Bhargava, *Smart Health Systems*,
https://doi.org/10.1007/978-981-16-4201-2_7

7.1 Necessity of CPSs

Human populations—and hence the numbers of patients requiring healthcare—are increasing exponentially. Many factors are responsible for poor human health, but the most important factor is ageing. Ageing comes with a variety of healthcare problems that cannot be ignored, and these problems require continuous and long-term medical care. CPSs can address these problems by keeping track of patients' health conditions continuously and even remotely, and sending the resulting data securely and easily to the relevant healthcare providers (see Fig. 7.1). Technological improvements in MCPSs ensure patient safety. With the ability to perform 24/7 monitoring of a patient without the need for any workforce or human intervention, it is very easy to collect data on the patient's condition. CPSs have the ability to integrate physical processes with computational communications, adding more intelligence to social life. The data that are gathered with the help of sensor devices can be easily articulated and warehoused on a server accessible to the relevant healthcare personnel. Medical data collected by medical sensors are very important for patient treatment, as they enable the ability to make treatment decisions; thus, it is necessary to make these data easy to access by the relevant medical personnel anywhere and at any time. Also, huge computational resources are needed by healthcare applications to perform efficient and smart decision making. Smart technologies and evolving predictive analytics are changing the healthcare environment [2].

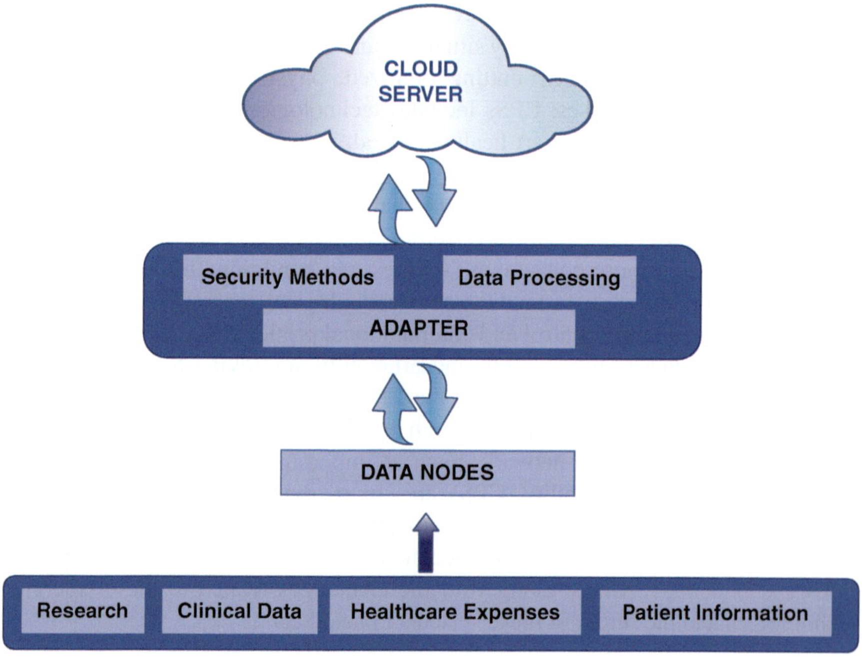

Fig. 7.1 Cyberphysical system for healthcare

CPSs integrated with various sensors can be used to collect information on patients and then transfer it to the cloud, which can use the power of computational methods to formulate results. The transferred data are secure enough to ensure that they cannot be manipulated to harm the patient instead of helping them. The decentralized nature of CPSs involves physical engineered systems in which all actions are well monitored, regulated, synchronized and securely combined by communication and computational techniques. Innovative CPS applications are gradually starting to function in societal spaces where humans play an important role. In the future, all applications utilizing CPSs will be more human centric.

Medical sensors can contribute to patient records, survivors can collect data on damage caused by natural disasters and drivers can provide information on traffic conditions in various locations. Typically, a CPS used in a social space can also be employed in a variety of healthcare programs through MCPSs [3]. Changes in the Internet and computers have opened up a vast set of new regulatory powers that can affect a person's health through mobility, new treatments, new energy management and new services. These are complex systems, connected to a network and integrated by different subsystems and cyberbody systems that integrate human communication as a central aspect [3]. CPSs can have a wide range of applications, such as intelligent medical technology, assisted living, environmental management and traffic management.

7.2 CPS Standards

This paradigm helps determine the essential constituents without needing to consider all possible instances, oversees the complexity involved and imposes order on it. The paradigm of CPSs can be grasped by considering on their three foundational constituents [4]:

1. The basic system framework
2. Knowledge and technical resources
3. Unique system attributes

The discipline of CPSs has already reached that stage of development, and regular traditional models have changed into the latest technological models, as described below.

7.2.1 Standard Model to Synergic Model

CPSs are an essential part of Information, Communications and Computational Technology (ICCT). The user interface creates a link between CPS technical environments and social environments.

Every system can be observed as an integrated structure of cybercomponents and physical components at all scales and levels [4]. The cybercomponents are distinct and logical, and they are responsible for computation, communication and control. In general, CPSs are interconnected in a synergic model. The model reflects ongoing progress with respect to the merging of both physical and cybertechnologies into one (i.e. the intersection between cybertechnologies and physical technologies as a new technology), and we refer to this technology as *synergic technology*. It performs fast and more efficiently than a traditional CPS.

7.2.2 Distinctive and Conceptual Realization Characteristics of CPSs

The paradigm of a cyberphysical system implies a set of different and distinctive characteristics. Implementation of CPSs has changed traditional processes in healthcare, and CPSs have great importance in modelling of newly equipped technologies in the system. The family of technologies includes [4]:

1. Abstraction and conceptual models
2. Logical frameworks and architectures
3. Functional and control models
4. Protocols and languages
5. Standards and regulations
6. Means of prototyping

The future models include purely mathematical models and information models of CPSs, which are based totally on multilevel abstraction and are termed *hybrid models*. The major challenges in CPSs are how to handle and format data in a structural way. Both logical and structural frameworks have proved to be important in conceptualizing CPSs [5]. The processing of CPSs is unified, synchronized, supervised and meticulous in computation, that may be distributed or clustered.

7.3 CPS Architecture

A healthcare CPS design can be framed on the basis of its infrastructure, such as a server-based or cloud-based infrastructure. A server-based infrastructure is ideal for minimal construction but requires individual maintenance. Recent operations have used a cloud-based infrastructure to measure cost effectiveness and accessibility. Given the complexity and limitations of resources, cyberobjects and physical objects can be vulnerable to a variety of challenges; therefore, special efforts are required when designing CPSs for health applications. In the healthcare sector, use of the cloud and big data not only is an important method but also is slowly becoming a new trend. Nowadays, medicine relies heavily on data collection and analysis, and as medical knowledge grows progressively, changes in the cloud and big data can have a profound impact on the healthcare industry, which has been transformed into a new biological system. That is why we need to create an appropriate health system to address the following challenges in this new transition [6].

Two major challenges in the architecture of CPSs are discussed below.

The design issues are as follows:

- *Multisource heterogeneous data management with unified standards:* These are needed to support scalability and to store the data efficiently.
- *Various data analysis modules with a unified programming interface:* An integrated system interface plays an important part in reducing system complexity and improving development and accessibility.
- *An application platform with a unified northbound interface:* In providing accessible and reliable health services, the application platform for the program is critical to resource utilization, technical support and information sharing.

The framework complexities are as follows:

- *The data collection layer:* This layer contains data nodes and adapters, providing an integrated interface for accessing data collected from multiple sources such as hospitals, the Internet and individual users.
- *The data management layer:* This layer has a distributed file storage (DFS) module and a compatible distributed parallel computing (DPC) module. With the help of big data–related technology, the DFS module improves the performance of the healthcare system by providing effective data storage and input/output (I/O) of healthcare data.
- *The application service layer:* This layer provides users with the basic results of visual data analysis. It also provides an integrated open application programming interface (API) for developers who intend user application to provide efficient, professional and personalized healthcare services.

7.4 Technologies Related to CPSs

Implementation of the physical components of CPSs—for example, sensors, actuators, transducers and transponders—needs advanced materials. While functionally supplemented materials and multifunctional materials represented real technological novelties a decade ago, carbon nanotubes, quantum dots, molecular switches, molecular motors etc. are now the focus of research. The reason is the revolution that is happening in science and technology, where efforts are being made to gain insights into the fundamental properties of material structures at the molecular scale.

There are even new research domains currently in formation, such as materiomics, which focuses on merging biology and engineering in sustainable and robust materials, and in multiscale molecular structures. These are not just strong and tough carbon-based materials but also next-generation self-learning material systems, whose properties can be tailored by changing their structures. Many kinds of advanced materials are already available for use in CPSs, such as peptide-based biomaterials, polymer-based biomaterials, ceramic based biomaterials, piezoelectric resources, shape memory alloys, electrorheological fluids and smart gels, polyethylene glycol, electro- and magnetostrictive materials, self-healing materials, electrochromic materials etc. Micromaterials with multilevel interior structures have been developed as a result of biomimetic and bioanalogy-inspired research. Examples of these are scaffolds and artificial skin.

The two main CPSs technologies on which we focus in this chapter are advances in macrorobotic technologies and synergic technologies.

7.4.1 Advances in Macro-robotic Technologies

The paradigm of advanced macrorobotics has developed rapidly in the last 40 years. Traditionally, macrorobotics has used principles and tools from solid mechanics, information technology and digital control [7].

The first-generation robots in the 1970s were immobile electromechanical devices with preprogrammed controls. The second generation of robots in the mid-1980s featured built-in sensors and articulated actuators. The third generation of robots built towards the end of the 1990s benefited from sophisticated computing and controlling software, which enabled smart reasoning, adaptiveness and context sensitivity. The currently studied and prototyped fourth-generation robots will have capabilities such as distributed architectures, situated communication, collaborative problem solving and autonomous decision-making. The fourth generation clearly shows a demarcation of macro- and mesoscale robotics versus micro-/nanosized robotics. This is reflected by our consideration of the branches of general robotic systems in our research and in this chapter. The paradigm of robots covers a wide range of device functionalities, implementations and applications. Mesoscale advanced robots are not just equipped with dextrous actuators, networked sensors, adaptive reasoning and learning; they are also intended to behave similarly to human beings. The current implementations range from industrial robots and automated guided vehicles (AGVs) thorough mobile domestic and service robots to smart humanoid and anthropomorphic (walking) robots [8]. In the context of CPSs, advanced robotics gives rise to new issues such as: (1) teleoperation and telerobotics, (2) increases in the functional intelligence of control systems, (3) neurocontrol of robotic devices and (4) unsupervised reasoning and learning by robots. The research aims to enable reverse engineering of the human brain in robots, which will give a completely different perspective to human–robot interactions [9].

7.4.2 Synergic Technologies

Interaction and cooperation are giving rise to a whole that is greater than the sum of single cyberphysical system technologies combined to make synergic technology. There are three main types of technologies in synergic technologies.

7.4.2.1 Digital Microchip Technologies

Conventional desktop and portable hardware designs, as well as current computing programs, are built on the premise that the principal task of a computer is sequential data transformation. However, there is an intrinsic demand for truly real-time information processing and large concurrency in CPSs [10]. This means that the principles of conventional computing have to be re-examined in the context of real-time collaborative CPSs, where the allowed time differences should be less than fragments of nanoseconds, given the operational characteristics (e.g. motion, contact etc.) of the physical components. The computing times should be reduced below the duration of the physical and cyberevents. This raises the need for even faster computing solutions and fuels efforts to create them. These are seen in various forms of particle-based computing that are currently at the boot-up stage. At this stage, particle-based computing research has discovered many more knowledge gaps and technological limitations than it has been able to resolve so far. It has also been conceived that as the configuration of the CPS computing platform changes as a result of upgrades or internal restructuring, the software should migrate to the incoming or changed devices and should adapt itself to the new objectives and functions. Research into computer-based computing is increasing and producing quantum computers that bind atoms and molecules to the work of processing, and remembering seems to be the next logical step. Quantum computers are capable of performing certain calculations much faster than any silicon-based computer can. They will also dissolve the boundaries between the cyber domain and the physical domain. Thanks to these and other current technological achievements, such as molecular sensors and nanoactuators, the difference between atoms and bits is disappearing. Similar trends are observable in the field of sensor technologies. Conventional instrument-type sensors are giving way to more versatile and effective sensor arrangements, substances and fields. Chemical, biological and nanotechnological research is producing new sensor solutions that require much less energy for their operation. The micro- and nanotechnology research of the near future will also go beyond the current embodiment and control principles of multiscale mechatronics-based systems, and this will change the world of micromachines and actuator technologies.

7.4.2.2 Sensor Network Technologies

One of the major functions of centralized or distributed CPSs is information distillation and control based on proactive operation of embedded sensor devices [11]. Sensors are rarely used alone; instead, they are used in clusters or networks. In these cases, the function of sensing is extended with signal conversion, transmission and communication. To control these, sensor manager agents are used that maintain a list of available sensors, processors, memories and switches, and provide access to them. Wireless sensor networks (WSNs) are typical manifestations of combined information-eliciting and transmission technologies [12]. In fact, WSNs are also typical from the perspective of issues related to the operation of transmitters at the network level. Common topologies are star and tree networks, but more flexible topologies are also possible at the cost of extra overheads and negotiation time. Depending on the tasks, the topology of the WSN and its synchronization can be adaptive. Data transmitted by the sensor nodes are collected, aggregated in memory and processed further in a master node or by dedicated host microprocessors. Signal transfer by transceivers may happen through wire-like transfer media or by wireless communication. In this respect, WSNs can be subdivided into preconfigured connection networks and broadcast-based networks. In heterogeneous sensor networks, signals are typically detected by various sensors at distributed locations, and the sensory data can be utilized by the sensors in multiple different modalities [13]. In the context of CPSs, sensors can also be seen as a branch of interfaces between the physical world and electronic signal processors. Modern sensors are already hardware and software combinations that can detect external events or environmental conditions on the basis of various principles. Such smart sensors provide information on (1) situations (the location, orientation, motion, image, lighting etc.), (2) physical attributes (humidity, temperature, pressure, force, light etc.) and (3) behavioural changes (mood, stress, haste, presence, proximity, gesture etc.). Logical sensors are also used to provide data without using a hardware device. In the case of many CPSs, an important issue is sensing crowd and collective human behaviour, collaborative system operations, complex social structures, or community-level phenomena and context. This makes the ability to collect, compare, filter and combine data from many users indispensable. Implementation of these functions, however, requires not just instrumentation but also efficient strategies for context-dependent interpretation, aggregation and operationalization of information [4].

7.4.2.3 Sub-microscale Electrochemical Technologies

As manifestations of CPSs, microsystems are appliances that are small, multifunctional and stand-alone but integrated. In general, they are built up from multiple microfabricated units and components, which enable their smart and integral behaviour (e.g. sensing, communication, reasoning and acting). There are three representative categories of microscale and submicroscale systems and technologies: (1) general microelectromechanical system (MEMS) technologies, (2) microrobotic technologies and (3) nanotechnologies. Originally produced on silicon wafers, MEMS devices have their roots in integrated circuits and semiconductors [14]. Current MEMS devices incorporate a comprehensive set of performance-enhancing technologies and integrate mechanical, sensory, actuator and electronic components into a standard substrate with microfabrication technology. The technologies used to create MEMS devices are generally classified as (1) surface micromachining, (2) bulk micromachining and (3) lithography, electroplating and melding (LIGA) technologies. Microgears, micropumps, micropipes, microrelays, micromirrors etc. are the typical devices produced by these technologies.

7.5 Benefits and Applications of CPS

CPSs comes with a whole lot of benefits, depending on the field in which they are applied. CPSs create a platform for solving real-time problems in the modern era. They allow for interrelation of different technologies such as distributed systems, real-time systems, control and monitoring systems, and wireless sensor-based networks. The revolutionary impacts of CPSs have been felt in different scopes of human life. They are widely deployed in areas such as healthcare, construction, smart buildings and cities, vehicles, manufacturing and energy management [1].

Some of the main areas of application of CPSs are discussed below.

7.5.1 Automobiles and Transportation

Conveyance of people and goods from one place to another is a very important necessity for human existence. The application of CPSs to the use of roads and highways to ensure the safety of road users is one defining point in the technological advancement of road safety. Another application of CPSs in the sphere of vehicle transportation is the model for optimization of system performance deployed for unmanned CPSs with wireless sensor network (WSN) movement. This primarily entails the vehicle receiving signals from the WSN for determination of movements and navigation. At times of emergencies, when promptness and timeliness are important, this aids navigation by paramedics to overcome obstructions such as traffic congestion. The integration of cybersystems with a conventional transportation system is known as a transportation cyberphysical system (TCPS). This is focused on monitoring, coordination and control of different modes of transportation. The constructs of a typical TCPS are the application, cyberspace and physical space. Cyberspace connotes the field where communications over networked computers occur, while the physical space refers to the physical presence in the real world. Creation of an intelligent transport system deploying a CPS involves effective combination of advanced sensors with embedded computational systems technology synchronized with cellular, wireless and satellite technologies for efficient management of traffic flow, safety assurance and project situation awareness [1].

7.5.2 Healthcare and Medicines

Improvement of digital technology has gone a long way towards enhancing healthcare delivery. From patients receiving treatment to medical personnel taking responsibility for administering medication, the ripples of technological advancement have been felt tremendously. With this advancement in technology, there are firm promises that in no time, patients' conditions can be assessed through CPSs even at different locations. Sensors in a CPS setup are built for collecting data related to the patient's health. Wireless communication serves as a medium for collecting the data via a gateway. The data gathered by the sensors are stored on a server and accessible to whoever needs them. There is an emphasis on data security, since patients' data are confidential. This is strictly adhered to in ensuring ethical and legal compliance. The development of CPSs for healthcare systems may be server based or cloud based. A supported server is ideal for small builds that require individual storage, whereas a cloud-based design allows for expansion, is cost effective and is easily accessible to large systems. As in other fields, CPSs require computational and communication processes to be carried out simultaneously. Depending on the application, identification of the system composition is done by the system architecture.

Much has been said about patients' health record details and privacy. The data stored in cloud storage and the subsequent information gained from them, is considered as the property of the patient. Restrictions are therefore placed on unwarranted acquisition of patients' health records or medical histories. Legal and ethical principles are strictly adhered to when CPSs are deployed in medical practice [1].

7.5.3 Manufacturing

The manufacturing sector has been a huge beneficiary of technological advancements over time. From the era of using crude and unsophisticated implements to the current era of the global virtual workforce, nanobased preventive maintenance, the Internet of Goods (IoG) and cloud computing, there has been a huge improvement in this sector. This sector's prominence in the economy of any nation has given it a relative advantage over other sectors. Manufacturing plays a pivotal role in the economic development of any country, particularly in developing countries. As production systems are becoming more complex, with ever-increasing demands from consumers for sophisticated goods, there is a need to rejig the processes and coordination of the assembly of different constituents making up the final end products. First, advanced communication allows real-time data acquisition from the physical world and the information response that comes through cyberspace. Second, intelligent data management analytics and computer capabilities create a cyberspace [1].

7.5.4 Security and Surveillance

Use of CPSs is firmly established in the area of security. Their application in this sphere has helped to curb crime and enable easy monitoring of private or public domains. One such application is the use of alarm systems. These systems establish a connection utilizing a cyberconnection through general packet radio codes with multiple accesses. With deployment of a mobile communications network, there is a synergy between communications control, terminal objects and users. The physical world is detected by the alarm using the terminal object, which is then connected to the users. In turn, the user can also control and monitor the physical world through transmission via an alarm communication system. This is one application of CPSs in security and surveillance defence units, and security departments of countries deploy CPSs to safeguard territorial landmarks. They are also used to monitor facilities and structures of national prominence. We must also not forget private security organizations commissioned to perform security duties for individuals and for public and private organizations. Such organizations deploy CPSs to perform their tasks for effective and smooth functioning.

7.5.5 Power and Thermal Energy Management

Access to power is a basic necessity for human existence, as almost all activities we carry out are linked to utilization of power. Industries are highly dependent on this sector for effective functioning. The banes of modern power grid systems are any factors that impinge on their reliability and efficiency. With the prominence of this sector being established, the needs to maintain infrastructural facilities and optimize the processes of power generation, transmission and distribution cannot be overemphasized. Over the years, assiduous efforts have been made in these areas. One such move is the application of CPSs in the processes of generation, transmission, management and consumption of power and thermal energy.

7.5.6 Smart Homes and Buildings

A model for use of CPSs with compatible architecture based on smart community architecture is called Networked Homes. A CPS is vital to fully realize the concept of the smart home. Activities such as controlling the heating system or the security apparatus, or deciding when to close the curtains or possibly switch on electronic devices are executed daily in homes. All of these can be performed with the modus operandi of a CPS. In such a setup, actuators and sensors are programmed to enable control via the Internet, which then aids the activities of the user through monitoring. Multifunctional sensors are incorporated into smart homes to measure physical features. Single units of smart homes collectively form what is termed a *smart community*. This is achieved with networking of smart homes to form a cluster, thereby fostering communal living. Single home units use multifunctional sensors, and human-controlled feedback is provided whenever it is required, improving home security and community protection.

7.5.7 Construction

The construction industry is infamous for being slow to embrace technological changes in its processes and procedures. This tendency has inhibited the industry from maximally leveraging the benefits that such advancements bring. However, recent studies have showcased the possibilities for infusing construction processes with CPSs. The *physical-to-cyber process* is a sensory process that involves sensor transmissions and other technologies to obtain information about building materials, and the *cyber-to-physical bridge* implies the actuation showing the effect of the sensed information on the system. In this context, actuation refers to control decisions based on the information gathered by the sensors so that construction activities, equipment and building components can be controlled.

7.6 CPSs for Healthcare (CPSsH)

With the rapid transformation of various medical systems, there is a marked need for new devices with increased performance. The term *medical cyberphysical systems* refers to programs that have a combination of embedded devices, software to control these devices and an interactive communication channel. Development of a safe and effective CPS for healthcare (CPSsH) requires new design, validation and testing strategies because of the increased size and complexity. The challenges of implementing these types of systems include clinical workflow, model-based development, close physical circulation, patient-specific algorithms, smart alarms, and design of a user-centred infrastructure for medical integration and collaboration. The nature of the CPSsH application ranges from patient monitoring to analgesic infusion pumps to inserted sensory devices. Cyberphysical modelling of the medical system and analysis of the proposed framework are performed to ensure the safety of the various applications. In one test, the condition that was considered was an analgesic infusion pump control algorithm for keeping the analgesic drug level in the blood within a certain limit [1]. This type of program is an example of systems that are often closed. Any change in the physical world can impact directly on the cyberworld, and action will be taken in the physical world on the basis of the instructions obtained from cyberspace [15].

The CPS structure offers a CPS development guide for industrial or medical applications. This structure has two main elements: (1) physical space and (2) cyberspace [16]. The structure shown in Fig. 7.2 provides a road map displaying the process used to build a CPS system from data acquisition to creative value. The structure contains smart connection, data-to-information conversion, and cyber, comprehension and communication levels.

7.7 CPSs Issues and Challenges

Many barriers prevent further design, development and implementation of cyber-physical systems in healthcare and other application areas. Designing a CPS for healthcare is a daunting task because it involves a number of issues such as software reliability, system interaction, computer intelligence, security and privacy, and contextual information. Software is an integral part of medical devices, and hardware functions in close collaboration with software.

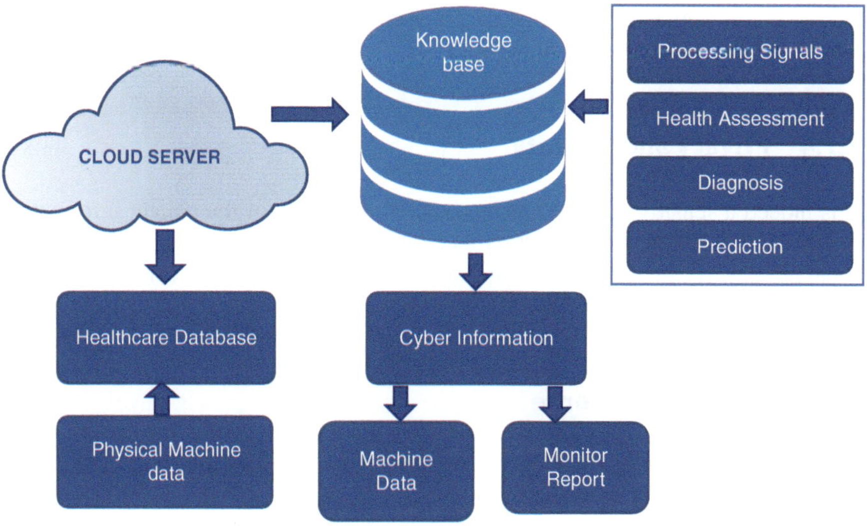

Fig. 7.2 Cyberphysical system (CPS) healthcare architecture

Major challenges and problems in healthcare [17] are discussed below.

7.7.1 Software Consistency

Software is an integral part of medical devices. Device performance and many functions are verified by software. The software also ensures that the interactions that occur between medical devices and patients are appropriate; therefore, the security and efficiency of the system depends on appropriate software development and management.

7.7.2 Medical Device Interactions

Many medical devices can have a variety of communication points. A well-maintained management system must be in place to integrate the various medical devices in a safe and secure way.

7.7.3 Data Mining

Medical equipment encounters many physical barriers in patients. The parameters are very different in nature and can provide not only general information about patients but also early predictions of future illness in order to prevent emergencies.

However, it is a challenging task to design such a system that can seamlessly remove complex physical barriers from patients.

7.7.4 Privacy and Security

It is indeed a sensitive task to ensure the confidentiality of the patient information that is collected. Unlawful use of patient data can result in identity and loss of personal privacy. It can also cause mental anguish and trauma, which can lead to development of physical illness.

7.7.5 Program Response

Response system development is a challenging task for CPSs in healthcare because the project will not be sustainable without a response system or patient care development. A CPS in a healthcare setting demonstrates a complete response system with a smart alarm system. The alarm system is very important to notify the caregiver of any possible illness or emergency. However, the alarm system needs to deal with specific challenges such as body parameter types, system complexity and start-up ability. It is important to choose the appropriate body parts to use when designing an alarm system.

7.7.6 Processing of Complex Queries

Because of the presence of different biosensors, use of wireless battery-powered sensors sometimes presents a number of limitations such as the need for low power consumption and limited operating power, which prevent the processor from processing complex questions. Complex questionnaire analysis can help reduce the amount of data transmission and speculation about the context. This functionality can reduce the power consumption of a limited power network. Complex questions can use access to many body parameters, thus predicting possible illness. However, this approach requires advanced design and computer skill sets.

7.7.7 Absence of a Prototype Structure

Currently, there is a shortage of safe and reliable architecture for testing and implementation of systems that include healthcare devices. For this reason, there has been failure to ensure the accuracy of CPSs in the construction of healthcare in an uncertain environment.

7.8 CPSs and Future Medical Devices

Use of CPSs can bring about radical change in the future of healthcare medical devices, as they unlock numerous new abilities to control medical resources to benefit human life. These CPS systems compose complex and hybrid integrated systems, which are being developed at an increasing rate. However, along with their positive aspects, there are some major challenges associated with CPSs and also many open issues that still need to be resolved on a CPS basis. Real-time communication support requires allocation of operating time for processor and network resources. A CPS can be considered a new IoT pattern with the expansion of WSNs, machine-to-machine (M2M) communication, radiofrequency identification (RFID), inevitable computer technology, network communication equipment and emerging control models. CPS applications have the advantage of benefiting from the largest smart devices and wireless networks that can handle CPS applications to deliver smart devices based on information from the mobile world. Therefore, one of the challenges is to provide the most effective CPS systems as a high-level IoT. Moreover, the next generation of CPS systems will not include the same computer models that are highly understandable and detemined. Finally, the most promising platform for healthcare systems includes IoT to enable healthcare reforms, protection of the interactive clinical environment with validation, and embedded, real-time and networked MCPSs. [18]

A description (map) of hyperphysical systems for healthcare applications has been presented, based on a complete taxonomy that includes eight different components: applications, buildings, range, data management, analysis, communication, security and control. These are complex, hybrid and network-connected systems integrated into different subsystems and cyberphysical systems that involve human communication as an integral part of them. This consideration applies to all modelling, including algorithm configuration, control areas, operation, implementation and maintenance. Therefore, the human factor needs to be analysed, understood and modelled. Cyberphysical systems mine another strand, where physical systems can be attacked in cyberspace by portable devices. Therefore, privacy and security are important to both the quality of life and the security of the economy. MCPSs deviate from the system's reliability rules in the event of errors. In physical systems, it is thought that many failures that occur immediately are impossible. Cyberattacks can be serious, revealing immediate or systematic failures. In general, a comprehensive approach to the real MCPS framework and the socio-cyberphysical system (SCPS) framework is essential. There is no integrated design approach to solve the challenges of designing and managing long-term learning outcomes and self-preparation for MCPSs. There is a wide gap between engineering technology and the development of high-end CPSs. To improve the situation, integration of knowledge of various interactions is essential. Cyberphysical systems should play a key role in building future engineering systems that are much more powerful than their current counterparts.

References

1. Ikuabe M, Aigbavboa C, Oke A (2020) Cyber-physical systems: matching up its application in the construction industry and other selected industries. In: Proceedings of the international conference on industrial engineering and operations management, Dubai, 10–12 Mar 2020, p 1543
2. Shi J, Wan J, Yan H, Suo H (2011) A survey of cyber physical systems. In: Proceedings of the 2011 international conference on wireless communications and signal processing (WCSP), Nanjing, 9–11 Nov 2011. https://doi.org/10.1109/WCSP.2011.6096958
3. Dey N, Ashour AS, Shi F, Fong SJ, Tavares JMR (2018) Medical cyber-physical systems: a survey. J Med Syst 42(4):74. https://doi.org/10.1007/s10916-018-0921-x
4. Horváth I, Gerritsen BH (2012) Cyber-physical systems: concepts, technologies and implementation principles. In: Proceedings of the ninth international symposium on tools and methods of competitive engineering, Karlsruhe, 7–11 May 2012, pp 19–36
5. Rajhans A, Cheng S-W, Schmerl B, Garlan D, Krogh BH, Agbi C, Bhave A (2009) An architectural approach to the design and analysis of cyber-physical systems. Electron Commun EASST:21. https://doi.org/10.14279/tuj.eceasst.21.286
6. Zhang Y, Qiu M, Tsai CW, Hassan MM, Alamri A (2015) Health-CPS: healthcare cyber-physical system assisted by cloud and big data. IEEE Syst J 11(1):88–95
7. Angeles J (2003) Fundamentals of robotic mechanical systems: theory, methods, and algorithms. Springer, New York
8. Cao YU, Fukunaga AS, Kahng AB (1997) Cooperative mobile robotics: antecedents and directions. Auton Robot 4:7–27
9. Egerstedt M (2000) Behavior based robotics using hybrid automata. In: Lynch N, Krogh B (eds) Hybrid systems: computation and control. Springer, New York, pp 103–116
10. Bell G, Dourish P (2007) Yesterday's tomorrows: notes on ubiquitous computing's dominant vision. Pers Ubiquit Comput 11:133–143
11. Wilson J (2008) "Sensor technology handbook", Newnes/Elsevier, Oxford, pp. 1–691
12. Chong C-Y, Kumar SP (2003) Sensor networks: evolution, opportunities, and challenges. Proc IEEE 91(8):1247–1256
13. Culler D, Estrin D, Srivastava M (2004) Guest editors' introduction: overview of sensor networks. Computer 37(8):41–49. https://doi.org/10.1109/MC.2004.93
14. Gardner JW, Varadan VK, Awadelkarim OO (2001) Microsensors, MEMS, and smart devices. Wiley, Chichester
15. Vijayaraghavan AW, Sobel A, Fox D, Dornfeld P, Warndorf P (2008) Improving machine tool interoperability using standardized interface protocols: MTConnect. In: Proceedings of the 2008 international symposium on flexible automation (ISFA), Atlanta, 23–26 Jun 2008
16. Petracca G, Sun Y, Jaeger T, Atamli A (2015) AuDroid: preventing attacks on audio channels in mobile devices. In: Proceedings of the 31st annual computer security applications conference, Los Angeles, 7–11 Dec 2015; pp 181–190. https://doi.org/10.1145/2818000.2818005
17. Haque SA, Aziz SM, Rahman M (2014) Review of cyber-physical system in healthcare. Int J Distrib Sens Netw 10(4):217415
18. Dey N, Ashour AS, Shi F, Fong SJ, Tavares JMR (2018) Medical cyber-physical systems: a survey. J Med Syst 42(4):1–13

Big Data Analytics and Cognitive Computing in Smart Health Systems

8

With advancements in technology in recent years, implementation of smart healthcare practices has increased. The data collected from patient treatment have been utilized to analyse health problem patterns in order to identify further similar cases. Big data analytics and cognitive computing are contributing considerable value to the healthcare system. The data volumes in the healthcare industry are massive and dynamic, with a great sense of complexity. Big data analytics and cognitive computing enable the healthcare system to store and formulate voluminous data for treating patients and computing uncertainty, with the help of existing databases. These intensive systems enhance healthcare systems and improve their efficiency in the existing environment [1]. A smart healthcare system requires a secure network infrastructure and cloud environments for advanced and reliable results. It will definitely require human intervention in most cases. In some general cases, patients can be treated with machine monitoring only at healthcare centres or hospitals. Elsewhere, the need to visit a hospital can be minimized and treatment of patients can be done online with help from some general monitoring equipment at the patient's home.

In this chapter, we discuss smart healthcare practices that use big data analytics and cognitive computing, and then adopt the results generated by these practices, further formulating the results and using them for treating patients.

The overview of electronic health records (EHRs) has changed healthcare systems dramatically. Evolution in an intelligent healthcare system takes a different approach to treating patients by making use of technologies such as big data analytics and cognitive computing. Big data analytics uses a completely different approach to the healthcare system, and there are data sets that are completely accessible to various organizations. The data spectrum in healthcare covers healthcare units, health insurers, health and medical researchers, government authorities, personal doctors, defence forces and so forth. Big data, as compared with traditional data, have an add-on advantage for the healthcare system, as they capture vast volumes of data on a patient, which are helpful in providing effective treatment in a short time [2]. Monitoring of the underlying disease and

S. Vyas, D. Bhargava, *Smart Health Systems*,
https://doi.org/10.1007/978-981-16-4201-2_8

measurements of the effectiveness of the patient's treatment can be analysed very efficiently with the help of big data. The analysis is done by machine learning and supervised learning algorithms. These algorithms play a vital role in treatment. Prediction and understanding of disease require cumulative analysis of the strong associations among the different systems in the patient's body, which thus includes combinations of the heart rate, blood flow rate, blood oxygenation rate and temperature in the initial phases of the diagnosis. After the initial diagnosis, the results that have been collected are formulated in order to select the appropriate treatment. Then cognitive computing, with the help of a machine learning algorithm, provides capabilities similar to human reasoning with the support of computational analysis by the machines. As shown in Fig. 8.1, there is a particular set of data that is utilized for cognitive computing: claims data, patient-generated data, clinical data, medical literature data, patient profile data and medical imaging data, all of which are computed to provide an outcome in the form of the suggested treatment.

As shown in Fig. 8.1, the different types of data (big data) are used to formulate probabilities in order to provide a recommendation and cognitive insights into the treatment [2]. Complex analysis and evaluation of the information are done in minimal time, then a comparison between the patient's data and the existing data pattern determines the appropriate treatment. Cognitive computing is regarded as a 'more human' type of artificial intelligence (AI).

This is a chance for big data analytics and cognitive computing to play vital roles in assisting the process of evaluation and availability, improving service delivery, assisting in the formulation and planning of health policy, providing comprehensive measurement methods, and evaluating complex and integrated healthcare data [3].

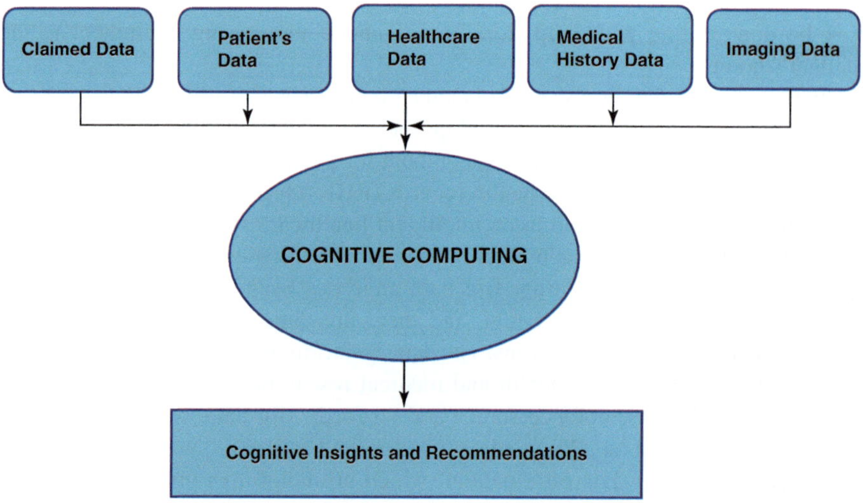

Fig. 8.1 Architecture for cognitive computing

8.1 Big Data Analytics

Data analytics is used to filter huge volumes of data in a very short period of time and to find treatment options and solutions for many important health problems. It can provide customized solutions on the basis of data sets gathered from individual patients. Big data analytics can improve outcomes on the basis of the patient's health information, provide personalized and advanced healthcare, and help to reduce medical errors [4]. Digitization and combination of data obtained from multiple consultants improves the quality of the healthcare system. The main advantage is the ability to detect disease at an early stage by analysing very few symptoms to prevent more serious illness in the patient. Big data analytics benefits healthcare by providing patient-centred and customized treatment as per the exact requirements, detection of disease with respect to underlying existing diseases, monitoring of the quality of the healthcare infrastructure, and improvements and advancements in treatment methods. Big data are accessible to facilities related to healthcare, including health management of individuals, disease observation, epidemic control, medical decision support etc.

8.1.1 Characteristics of Big Data

- *Heterogeneousness:* In healthcare, big data can be classified into two formats: structured and unstructured data. The EHR gathers structured data, which are organized with human intervention. However, most healthcare data are unstructured. The sources of data include data from individual patients' laboratory tests and computed tomography (CT), magnetic resonance imaging (MRI), and X-ray examinations. There is still a shortage of available tools for analysis of unstructured data that require human intervention.
- *Incompleteness:* Real-time data from monitoring devices recording changes in a patient's body are generally not stored in healthcare records and hence cannot be included in analyses with other data. because it is not useful to store complete data sets of this type. However, improving the Healthcare records support patient care, medical audits, epidemiology, medical research and resource sharing [5]. These data always remain incomplete when they are analysed as big data completeness of the data with the help of machine learning algorithms and collection of results-oriented data sets can improve healthcare quality.
- *Timeliness and longevity:* Diagnostic examinations such as electrocardiography (ECG), single-photon emission computed tomography (SPECT) and MRI include a time function and therefore have accurate timing [5]. The storage time of diverse medical actions like storing one patient's data for multiple diagnostics becomes difficult to record; therefore, it is useful to know the patient's history to support decision making about the most appropriate treatment.
- *Data privacy:* Privacy of patients' personal and medical data stored by healthcare providers is essential. Centralization of the storage of data should be safe and secure but can be vulnerable to cyberattacks, which can cause great harm to both patients

and healthcare organizations. Personal healthcare applications that collect data on an individual person (e.g. fitness bands, Google Fit and other fitness-tracking applications) provide an idea of the person's physical health but also entail a degree of control over the person. Hence, big data or cloud data must be kept secure and accessible only to authenticated persons in order to avoid misuse of the data.

- *Ownership:* Big data deals with various patient's cases like a consumer having medical needs and also verify these details but again this is not applicable to all the details of a patient. Other vital information is stored and managed by hospitals, doctors, laboratories, dispensaries and government organizations, to which consumers lack access for managing their data. Use of big data can enable patients to have access to all of their own health data so it can be used wherever and whenever it is required, even remotely.

8.1.2 The 'Four V's' of Big Data Analytics in Healthcare

As time goes on, there will be continuous generation and accumulation of healthcare data, which may result in unbelievably huge volumes of data being collected at increasing velocity, in different varieties and with different levels of veracity as to the degree of their usefulness. These are known as the 'four V's' of big data analytics in healthcare (Fig. 8.2), the main features of which are discussed below.

- *Volume:* The concept of big data refers to collection and handling of large volumes of data. There is no volume limit for these data. In this context, volume refers to the huge multitude of heterogenous data that must be organized, maintained and analysed to treat patients and further improve healthcare services [6].
- *Velocity:* This refers to the speed of big data collection by smart healthcare devices. The growth of data is increasing continuously. To analyse the impact of

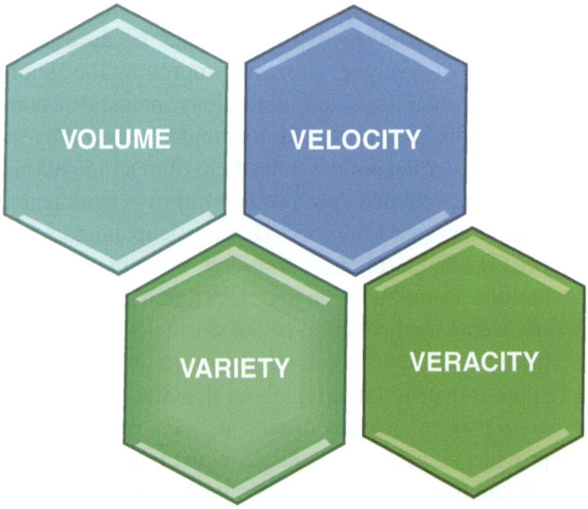

Fig. 8.2 The 'four V's' of big data in healthcare

this growth on healthcare services, it is very important to keep track of the velocity of the data growth [6].

- *Variety:* Big data are composed of various types of data—mainly structured and unstructured data, which can be textual, visual, audible or sensor-based data. Structured data include medical data, which must be collected, deposited and managed. The generated structured data comprise EHR healthcare data. Unstructured and semistructured data include e-mails, photographs, video and audio recordings, and a variety of healthcare-related information such as clinical reports, prescriptions, and X-ray imaging [7].
- *Veracity:* Data veracity is a level of data compatibility assurance. Various data sources differ in terms of their data integrity and reliability. The results of big data analytics should be reliable and error-free, but in healthcare, machine learning algorithms could potentially make automated decisions on the basis of data that were useless or misleading [7].

8.1.3 Architecture of Big Data Analytics in Healthcare

The big data framework in healthcare is similar to traditional data storage techniques. However, the key variance—or, say, the main benefit of big data analytics—is data processing achieved by use of different analytical methods and tools to formulate the massive volumes of data into useful results. The big data analytics framework is based on a distributed computer system, which enables fast processing of results from different sources of input. After collection, transformation of the data takes place. The architecture of big data is very complex, but it refines unstructured and structured data into simpler data sets, which are further used for treatment of diseases in healthcare (Fig. 8.3).

The framework consists of a data source layer, data transformation layer, platform layer and analytics application layer. The data source layer is basically focused on internal and external resources related to healthcare data collected from various locations and in different formats. The transformation layer is in charge of functions such as mining, translation, and uploading of data to the big data framework, using a variety of data production methods such as middleware and data storage processes. The big data platform layer has a variety of Hadoop tools that perform certain functions on the Hadoop distributed file system (HDFS), utilizing the MapReduce system model. The analytics application layer accomplishes functions such as query execution, reporting, online processing and data-mining techniques.

8.1.4 Process of Big Data Analytics

Big data analytics works with several processes, which include data collection, data processing, data cleaning and data analysis. These steps are carried out to analyse huge data sets in order to facilitate organization for efficient processing of the data [8].

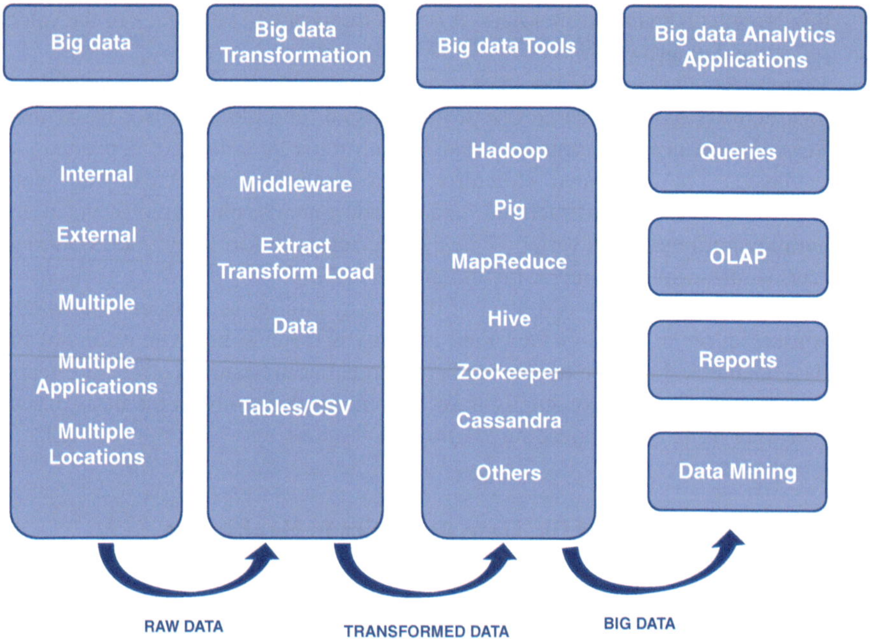

Fig. 8.3 Basic architecture of big data analytics. *CSV* comma-separated values, *OLAP* online analytical processing

8.1.4.1 Phases of Big Data Processing

- *Data collection:* Collection of healthcare data is the most important factor in prescription of appropriate treatments for patients. Structured and unstructured data are collected from various sources—such as the cloud, sensors and Internet of Things (IoT) devices—and deposited in a data warehouse.
- *Data processing:* After collection of the data, they are organized appropriately to formulate the results. The organized and stored data are processed using two main processing techniques:
  - Batch processing for large data volumes
  - Stream processing for fast processing of small data volumes
- *Data cleaning:* After formulation of the data (and depending on whether the data volume is small or large), the first requirement of the analytics process is to clean the data by formatting it properly and removing redundancies or irrelevant data sets to improve the quality of the data.
- *Data analysis:* This is the final phase in the process and puts the data into a useful format. The techniques used in data analytics are:
  - Deep learning to discover data patterns and produce the desired results; use of algorithms based on AI and machine learning is required.
  - Data mining, which involves arrangement of useful data from the raw data and classification of the data to improve the capacity to search the data in a variety of data sets.

- Predictive analysis to predict outcomes or results before any real-time activity occurs, in order to minimize and avoid uncertainty and risks.

8.1.5 Need for Big Data in Healthcare

Use of big data enables rapid analysis of huge volumes of data, which can result in better care for patients in an efficient way. Big data analytics is important for healthcare systems because it utilizes vast volumes of data from multiple sources in various formats in order to recognize opportunities and allow physicians to act faster and provide effective treatment. Big data analytics serves as a cost-saving model by identifying multiple options for treatment from multiple sources of information. Adoption of different methodologies can provide better understanding of the physical and mental health status of a patient through collection of different data sets. Healthcare analytics actually helps to reduce medical costs, predict epidemic outbreaks, prevent diseases, and improve quality of life. Use of big data to create health strategic plans for the future is the most important advantage of data analytics. It can also reduce fraud and human errors, enhancing the data security of the healthcare system. There is now a trend towards greater patient involvement in data collection to maximize the available data on patients and send alerts to their healthcare providers in order to avoid potential health problems.

8.1.6 Big Data Framework for Smart Healthcare

Big data healthcare analytics is related to the execution of computer programs. In a conventional system, healthcare relies on other organizations for big data analysis. Many healthcare participants rely on information technology providers because they can achieve remarkable results and their operating systems' performance is efficient and can process varied data into similar forms. Nowadays, however, healthcare systems face many challenges in attempting to quickly implement big data–based healthcare. The use of big data is increasing and has the potential to provide important information of great relevance to healthcare systems. As mentioned above, the large volumes of generated data are deposited in the form of hard copies, which are then transformed digitally [7].

The frameworks for healthcare data analysis are:

- *Predictive analytics:* Big data analytics involves numerous methods, including text analytics and multimedia analytics, though the most important method is predictive analytics. It incorporates arithmetical approaches such as mining and machine learning techniques, which are helpful for storage of current and past data for use in future predictions. Predictive analytics procedures are now utilized in healthcare systems to identify at-risk patients.
- *Machine learning:* The concept of machine learning is very similar to that of data mining. Machine learning recognizes data patterns and consequently modifies

programming methods. Instead of mining data on the basis of personal understanding, machine learning utilizes the data to advance the program's understanding.
- *eHealth records:* This is the most comprehensive healthcare data application that utilizes big data. Each patient has his or her own medical reports, including details of their health history, any allergies, symptoms and test outcomes. These files are flexible because doctors can easily update them from time to time and add new health test results without the need for paperwork or data retrieval.

8.1.7 Big Data Applications for Healthcare

- Big data medical image analysis
- Medical signal analytics
- Genomics related to big data applications
- Patient predictions for service improvement
- Health data using expert strategic planning
- Prediction analysis in healthcare
- Minimization of fraud and strengthening of security
- Integration of big data and medical imaging
- Smart human resource management
- Smart risk and healthcare management
- Advanced asset management
- Smart techniques for therapies and medications

8.2 Cognitive Computing for Healthcare

Cognition is a summary of the thought methods people use to communicate with others and the environment. It is often defined as a system of cognitive functions ranging from visual perception to social comprehension. Cognitive systems in healthcare have powerful features due to the latest developments in traditional AI with the discovery of new technologies, rapid advancement of new machine learning techniques and greater data acquisition from a set of different resource devices. Developments in medicine are occurring rapidly, but the cognitive impacts of numerous diseases have not been addressed adequately [9]. Cognitive computing depends on knowledge only; in real communication, the details are mostly represented by data, including formal and informal data. Essentially, cognitive computing utilizes computer-based models to mimic the process of human thought in adverse situations where the answers may be vague and indeterminate [10].

Big data analysis and cognitive computing differ in terms of data volume, though both provide efficient solutions. Cognitive computing has great utility for both academic and healthcare projects. Cognitive computing offers an efficient way for a machine to identify a patient's requirements and allows it to provide deeper insight into human cognition in order to provide an intelligent cognitive service for the user [11]. The proliferation of computer technology and rapid advancements in semantics, information theory and data science are bringing about remarkable and thought-provoking cognitive changes.

Problem solving by machines is possible only because they use cognitive methods in a way similar to the simulations performed during analysis processes, which are similar to human thinking. The results produced by the simulations can be correct and very close to those resulting from live decision-making by humans. However, the main difference is that cognitive computing relies on the machine and supervised learning algorithms, which can also yield unexpected results in real-life situations, such as in healthcare. Thus, it can contribute to smart healthcare system at a very basic level when used with human interventions.

8.2.1 Cognitive Analytics Architecture

Cognitive computing is purely based on specific technologies such as fifth-generation cellular wireless networks (5G), robotics, deep learning, machine learning and IoT or cloud technologies. The framework supports health supervision, cognitive healthcare and smart healthcare. Cognitive computing involves very complex architecture and thus requires a lot of information to produce the expected results. The results are based only on the input provided by humans, which can be in the form of massive volumes of data.

The framework of cognitive computing comprises three main technologies:

- *Internet of Things (IoT):* IoT collects diverse real-time and valuable information from different sensors and other healthcare objects used in the healthcare infrastructure. IoT involves perception and transmission of information. Widespread use of IoT will produce huge volumes of data and be a significant source of information for understanding cognitive computing. Also, as a new kind of computing mode, cognitive computing will provide ways to practise with better efficiency, visual perception and data gathering in IoT.
- *Big data analytics:* The continuing rise in data collection and the continuous improvement in computing power are proving to be irreplaceable in the era of big data. Cognitive computing requires a simpler and more suitable method than big data analysis. The rise of AI and the support of cloud resources offer the benefits of cognitive computing developments.
- *Cloud computing:* Cloud computing makes computation, storage and bandwidth widely available. Therefore, it cuts the cost of deploying software services and offers industrial support and advancement of cognitive computing applications. For generation of large volumes of real-life data, after big data analysis is performed in the cloud computing framework, technologies such as machine learning are implemented for data mining and applying its results in various fields.

Cloud computing and IoT offer a basis for software and hardware related to cognitive computing. On the other hand, big data analytics provides approaches and assumptions to discover and identify new advancements and values of data [11].

8.3 Healthcare and Data Management Role Players

The different players involved in healthcare data management roles are listed below [12]. The data accessible to these different players are shown in Fig. 8.4.

- *Patients:* They generate healthcare data such as personal identification data, test analyses and past medical history in a nondigital format.
- *Healthcare workers:* Individuals or firms offer health services and generate (1) patient medical accounts, (2) information from medical sensor devices, (3) hospital admission records, (4) medical textbooks, (5) medical journals, (6) research studies, (7) regulation reports, (8) bills, and (9) cost data.
- *Pharmaceutical companies:* They manage data supporting pharmaceutical research, clinical trials and drug effectiveness, and prescriptions from healthcare providers.
- *Healthcare financiers:* These are organizations that raise funds for healthcare work (including insurance firms, remote employers, government and the public) and generate information related to billing and service reviews.
- *Government administrative services:* They generate regulatory information.
- *Healthcare information providers:* They generate data on the usage and efficacy of prescription medicines, health terminology classifications and software solutions for healthcare data analysis.
- *Healthcare information facilities:* These are individuals or firms that provide healthcare guidance or reports for improvements in the healthcare community.

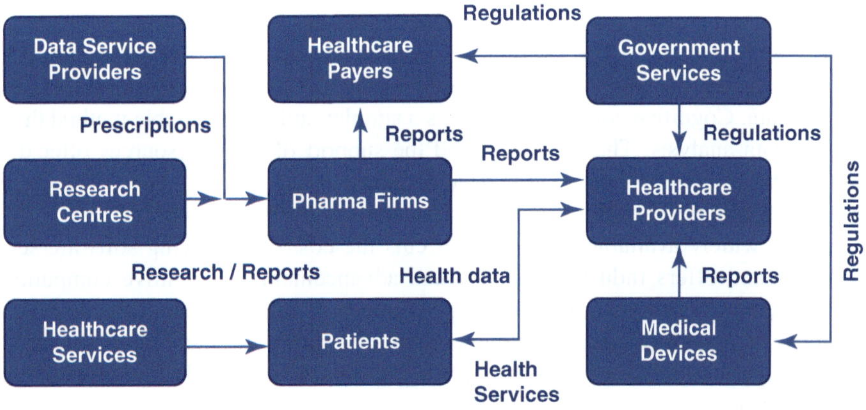

Fig. 8.4 Data accessible to different players in healthcare data management

- *Health research centres:* These are teams of researchers working on or leading independent research, developing healthcare projects on a diversity of topics, and producing research and reporting data.
- *Healthcare device makers:* They generate research reports and data. The identified patient information can be categorized into profiles: (1) a main profile, (2) a health profile, (3) a routine profile and (4) a social profile with full records. This confines the information that can be accessed by the system and results in an incomplete medical record.

8.4 Impact of Cognitive Computing Systems on Healthcare

Cognitive computing systems use a variety of data capture methods involving litigation, patient-centred data, clinical data, medical literature, patient profiles and medical opinion. After due consideration, they provide insights and potential recommendations. The main impacts of utilizing such systems are as follows [12]:

- Communication of timely insights to individuals
- Identification of at-risk patients
- Prediction of patient health and costings
- Support for self-medication and treatment decisions
- Endorsement of interventions based on opportunities for success
- Improvement of patient engagement and communication by use of technologies such as mHealth and wearable sensor apps
- (With use of natural language processing (NLP) technology) linking of relevant clinical studies and information-driven help with data processing
- Assistance for researchers to understand genomic data
- Assistance for researchers to link pathogens to many of the natural and human factors that affect human health
- Guidance for physicians to provide precision medication for each patient
- Incorporation of advanced image and text processing
- Development of intensive care unit (ICU) data systems and integration of portable monitoring data with EHRs
- Development of a forecasting model for identifying health risks and financial risk management
- Help for patients to develop services with customized information and community support
- Conversion of unstructured documents into structured data

8.5 Smart Healthcare Approaches

- Advanced machine learning and reinforcement learning
- Knowledge-based approaches
- Deep learning

- Real-time analytics
- Clinical reasoning
- End user–driven data analytics
- NLP and text analytics
- Healthcare knowledge-bases
- High-performance genome analysis
- Understanding and reliability in analytics

8.6 Big Data Challenges in Healthcare Systems

These challenges include the following [13]:

- *Data processing–related challenges:* Analysis of massive volumes of data
- *Manpower-related challenges:* Availability of skilled persons to operate machines
- *Domain-related challenges:* Dynamic technologies to use in order to work in multiple domains at the same time
- *Managerial and organizational challenges:* Management of an organization as a whole system to work efficiently and produce reliable results

Some challenges that will always persist in smart healthcare systems are:

- Security and privacy
- Data quality
- Integration of heterogeneous data sets
- Lack of static values related to healthcare

8.7 Big Data and Cognitive Technology Future Plans for Healthcare

Healthcare strategies are struggling to provide better customer care, service and satisfaction, and to operate with better understanding in the midst of tough competition even while focusing on reduction of costs [14].

- *Marketing strategies:* Market analysis can be performed using the collected data sets, and plans can be made to implement cognitive technologies for optimal interpretation of big data.
- *Development and maintenance of networks:* Big data with machine learning algorithms are creating a more healthy environment between patients and healthcare infrastructures by minimizing fraud through implementation of cognitive computing for fraud detection.

- *Risk management:* Cognitive computing plays a significant part in the development of value-added healthcare systems. This demands a systematic understanding of costs incurred and healthcare results related to healthcare systems [14].
- *Sales:* Sales definitely increase with progressive analytical methods, machine learning techniques, and utilization of automatic tools to help consumers choose the most appropriate healthcare plans.
- *Patient engagement:* The patient data collected using different devices at healthcare centres can improve efficiency through analysis of the records and results generated by the devices. Formulation of big data followed by use of cognitive computing for decision-making on the basis of the data sets will always provide advantages for smart healthcare systems.

This chapter has discussed the various positive aspects and challenges for smart healthcare systems posed by the advancement of technologies and implementation of cognitive computing to make smart healthcare systems more efficient with formulation of data sets from big data. It has also discussed big data and cognitive computing aspects relevant to healthcare, along with their challenges and future developments. However, more advancements are still awaited in this field.

References

1. Coccoli M, Maresca P (2018) Adopting cognitive computing solutions in healthcare. J E-Learn Knowl Soc 14(1):57–69. https://doi.org/10.20368/1971-8829/1451
2. Behera RK, Bala PK, Dhir A (2019) The emerging role of cognitive computing in healthcare: a systematic literature review. Int J Med Inform 129:154–166
3. Belle A, Thiagarajan R, Soroushmehr SM, Navidi F, Beard DA, Najarian K (2015) Big data analytics in healthcare. Biomed Res Int 2015:370194. https://doi.org/10.1155/2015/370194
4. Wang L, Alexander CA (2019) Big data analytics in healthcare systems. Int J Math Eng Manag Sci 4:17–26. https://doi.org/10.33889/IJMEMS.2019.4.1-002
5. Liang H, Luo M, Wang R, Lu P, Lu W, Long L (2018) Big data in health care: applications and challenges. Data Inform Manag 2(3):175–197. https://doi.org/10.2478/dim-2018-0014
6. Hitachi (2021) Big data. https://social-innovation.hitachi/en-in/knowledge-hub/collaborate/big-data. Accessed 20/3/2021
7. Kumar S, Singh M (2018) Big data analytics for healthcare industry: impact, applications, and tools. Big Data Mining Anal 2(1):48–57. https://doi.org/10.26599/BDMA.2018.9020031
8. Tableau (2021) Big data analytics: what it is, how it works, benefits, and challenges. https://www.tableau.com/learn/articles/big-data-analytics#:~:text=Big%20data%20analytics%20describes%20the,the%20help%20of%20newer%20tools. Accessed on 25/03/2021
9. Wallin A, Kettunen P, Johansson PM, Jonsdottir IH, Nilsson C, Nilsson M, Eckerström M, Nordlund A, Nyberg L, Sunnerhagen KS, Svensson J, Terzis B, Wahlund LO, Kuhn GH (2018) Cognitive medicine—a new approach in health care science. BMC Psychiatry 18(1):42. https://doi.org/10.1186/s12888-018-1615-0
10. Botelho B (2018) Cognitive computing. TechTarget. https://searchenterpriseai.techtarget.com/definition/cognitive-computing#:~:text=Cognitive%20computing%20is%20the%20use,IBM's%20cognitive%20computer%20system%2C%20Watson. Accessed on 18/02/2021
11. Chen M, Herrera F, Hwang K (2018) Cognitive computing: architecture, technologies and intelligent applications. IEEE Access 6:19774–19783. https://doi.org/10.1109/ACCESS.2018.2791469

12. Ogiela MR, You I, Yim K (2013) Cognitive and secure computing in information management. Int J Inf Manag 33(2):243–244
13. Mehta N, Pandit A (2018) Concurrence of big data analytics and healthcare: a systematic review. Int J Med Inform 114:57–65
14. Schatsky D, Petrov P, Ronanki R (2015) Cognitive technologies for health plans: using artificial intelligence to meet market demands. Deloitte. https://www2.deloitte.com/content/dam/insights/us/articles/artificial-intelligence-health-plans/DUP_1087-Cognitive-Technologies_Health-Plans_MASTER.pdf. Accessed on 30/11/2020

9 Values and Risks Associated with Smart Health

The recent evolution of healthcare systems has enhanced the overall experience of smart health by creating an infrastructure equipped with smart devices. Smart healthcare devices make crucial and valuable contributions in health monitoring and diagnostics. Smart health is all about tracking and monitoring the health status of the patient with use of smart devices. The information collected from these devices needs to be reliable, secure and based on real-time measurements. A critical problem for a healthcare system is that it has fewer remedial amenities for the purpose of tracking a patient's past history, which can be quite helpful for providing an actual cure. Thus, it is necessary to optimize the overall health system by implementing smart healthcare practices. Optimized systems can provide more accurate diagnoses and can monitor the condition of the patient with transparency. The changes that occur continuously in the human body require real-time interpretation. Medical researchers, healthcare scientists and biologists are continuously working to improve predictive algorithms for smart healthcare to minimize the risks of severe health problems developing. Smart health solutions provide efficient monitoring of specific factors such as the blood pressure, blood oxygen and sugar levels, the heart rate and body temperature, which do not require a doctor's specific attention in normal cases. Smart healthcare aids the purpose of exploiting accessible resources to their full potential [1]. The response time of smart healthcare is very short, as it can analyse the body's activities over a brief period and generate alerts about the person's health status. However, along with all of these advantages and values, there are enormous challenges in smart health that can increase risks. The complete realization on the sensor-based results may risk to the patient but in least cases. The responsibility involved in creating these devices is huge because any malfunctions can have important adverse consequences. These connected technologies enable healthcare facilities to operate remotely when there is a need for assistance from a healthcare professional. Security breaches involving patients' data can make them very vulnerable; for example, inappropriate use of personal data can put a patient or their family at very high risk.

S. Vyas, D. Bhargava, *Smart Health Systems*,
https://doi.org/10.1007/978-981-16-4201-2_9

This chapter examines the value and risks associated with smart health. It also identifies factors that are important in keeping a smart healthcare system efficient, reliable and secure. Smart healthcare systems serve the needs of human beings in two ways: either through monitoring at home with use of basic gadgets or through treatment in healthcare facilities with more advanced tools. Smart health expertise adds value for citizens, healthcare workforces and indeed the whole of humanity.

- *Primary recognition and intervention:* Early detection can cure many diseases at a very early stage and reduce the risk of developing more severe conditions. The intervention of a healthcare professional on the basis of the patient's health status can determine the appropriate treatment for the patient. Detection of an underlying disease and its effects on other primary diseases can avoid exacerbation of the situation. If all necessary steps are taken, including precautions or treatment, hospitalization of the patient can possibly be avoided.
- *Personalized treatment:* The treatment given to any patient with any problem is generalized in the early phases. When the cause is identified, and if the problem persists, extra actions are taken. However, with the help of smart healthcare devices, the problem can be treated using targeted solutions. Treatment that is personalized in accordance with the initial health status of the patient can shorten their recovery time.
- *Improved healthcare processes and patient journeys:* Implementation of smart healthcare improves the quality and processes involved in the healthcare system. It expedites the process of treatment with efficient and reliable results. There is less need for patients to visit a hospital than in a traditional healthcare system. Electronic health records (EHRs) and diagnostic systems can produce results digitally and quickly so that more patients can be treated in minimal time. The facilities that are provided, such as digital reports and digital assessment of the patient's problem, improve the quality of the patient's journey in the healthcare system.

Nonetheless, there are some caveats that need to be considered:

- *Necessity of social and organizational transformation:* The latest technology is an advancement of traditional technology but requires an infrastructure in which smart healthcare devices can be installed. The compatibility of existing devices with new and advanced devices is one of the biggest challenges. A conducive work culture and cooperation from skilled healthcare professionals to operate or manage the devices are crucial.
- *Reliability of continuous monitoring:* The accuracy of continuous monitoring by smart healthcare devices is unproven [2]. There can be many reasons behind uncertainty of monitoring results—for example, system failure in a machine, device incompatibility, power cuts or internal interruptions. These factors can easily skew the results.
- *Safety and security of personal information:* Data on healthcare centres, healthcare workers, healthcare professionals and patients can be very vulnerable if

hacking or unauthorized access occurs. Data breaches can potentially harm the healthcare system. Patient data can be compromised and used in illicit ways to harm the patient. It is vital that security checks are performed routinely on all data associated with the system.

9.1 Goals of Smart Health Systems

Smart health systems involve restructuring of healthcare systems to provide better care, improve treatment outcomes, reduce patients' costs, improve procedures and workflows, and provide a better-quality patient experience of healthcare services [3].

The major goals of a smart health system are:

- *Cost reductions:* A smart health-monitoring system monitors patient health conditions in real time and can therefore reduce unnecessary appointments with doctors, hospitalizations and therefore also expenditure.
- *Efficient and improved treatment:* Physicians' decisions can be more evidence based, ensuring complete transparency in health monitoring.
- *More effective and faster diagnosis of disease:* Continuous patient monitoring and use of real-time data allow illness to be detected in a very early phase, or a precursor to that illness can be sensed in time to prevent it. Determination of an underlying disease can expedite its diagnosis and treatment.
- *Proactive treatment:* Consistent monitoring of patient health with the help of smart equipment provides opportunities for proactive treatment.
- *Medical and smart device management:* One of the critical challenges for the healthcare industry is management of smart devices and medicines. Use of connected devices allows them to be managed appropriately and cost effectively.
- *Reductions in errors:* Data generated by smart healthcare devices are helpful for decision-making and help to ensure that healthcare processes operate smoothly with fewer errors and at lower cost.

Implementation of data safety procedures is essential. Smart healthcare reconnoitres novel investigation in terms of patient cure via real-time or dynamic health nursing.

There are three aims for a smart healthcare framework [4]:

- *Refining the quality of nursing care:* Improved and advanced facilities can be provided for patients, and digital patient monitoring can give a better idea of how long the treatment will take. This creates a positive mindset for the patient and a ray of hope, which supports the patient mentally.
- *Improving patient outcomes:* Feedback and input from the patient play a decisive role in patient treatment.
- *Reducing the cost of care:* Computerized monitoring systems can take care of patients more effectively than humans, as they produce results of diagnostics in a digitized format, which gives a better idea of the patient's health status.

9.2 Principles of Smart Health Systems

- *Efficacy:* Smart healthcare systems need to be efficient in terms of energy consumption, as they depend on devices positioned on different body parts to obtain health information on the user. If a healthcare device runs out of battery power every now and then or requires exterior energy resources, the practical implementation of the system is negatively affected [5]. To ensure efficiency, each device's operational status should be maintained, with regular checks of the performance of the device, and they should be repaired, upgraded or replaced when needed.
- *Quality improvement:* The increase in the population has increased demands for healthcare facilities. It is a very big challenge to maintain the quality of treatment for everyone. However, lack of access to appropriate healthcare can result in infections turning into illness outbreaks, and these, in turn, can result in epidemics and necessitate containment zones, which are costly to implement [6]. Quality improvement in healthcare can be achieved with smart healthcare systems through remote monitoring by specialists and treatment by advanced smart devices that can be deployed wherever they are required. Accurate diagnosis of disease by smart devices is another advantage of a smart healthcare system.
- *Attention to personal data:* Privacy of personal data and data on healthcare systems is very important. Relevant personal data need to be available to the appropriate persons when needed but otherwise kept secure. The same applies to data on clinical and diagnostic processes, which can facilitate achievement of objectives with a minimal error rate, high accuracy and cost effectiveness, with access to internal and external resources whenever desirable [7].
- *Expansion of patient capabilities:* New developments in mobile and microelectronic health-monitoring technology are transforming the roles of both doctors and patients in modern healthcare systems. However, the incorporation of this technology into medical practice is still limited [8]. Patients' capabilities are enhanced by use of reliable smart devices, wearables and sensors, which can play a preventive role in many health conditions.
- *Relationships between patients and medical organizations:* The relationships between healthcare organizations and patients are improved when patients trust and have confidence in doctors and other healthcare workers. Transparency regarding healthcare expenses and results-based diagnostics helps to create heathy relationships between medical organizations and patients.
- *Professional development through information technology:* Information technology has revolutionized healthcare practices by introducing major developments in healthcare and advances in continuing professional education of healthcare workers.
- *Safe data exchange:* Data security is determined by the security protocols used in networks and algorithms that are implemented in servers for data exchange.

- *Expansion of the healthcare framework:* The healthcare framework is becoming smarter and broader with the introduction of smart health. This has opened up various opportunities for healthcare professionals and the whole healthcare system.
- *Ethical standards:* Individual medical information may be quite helpful in providing valued and significant individual benefits for medical research purposes. However, disclosure of this information could have an adverse impact on society as a whole if it were wrongly presented and interpreted. This kind of unsuitable use of information infringes the moral ethics of medical practice [9].
- *Accessibility for everyone:* A smart healthcare system should be universal and hence accessible to everyone in the world with certain validations according to the relevant categories, such as doctors, patients, healthcare centre staff etc.

9.3 Classification of Smart Healthcare

One of the chief objectives of smart healthcare is to help users by informing them of their health status and making them conscious of their health. Smart healthcare systems make users able to self-manage and track their health, and to utilize applications (apps) that perform functions such as calorie counting, step monitoring etc. Smart healthcare includes operations that are totally independent, as well as others that can help users to obtain advice from healthcare specialists. The rudimentary architecture of a smart healthcare structure is shown in Fig. 9.1 [1].

This smart healthcare structure is centred on the functions performed by medical hardware devices, the relevant technologies, the applications used and the system administration, in addition to the end users. Connectivity technology plays a vital role in expansion of the applications that the healthcare system is designed for. All of these together form a complete smart healthcare system.

9.4 Smart Health System Essentials

The following are essential parts of a smart healthcare system [1]:

- *Requirements in smart healthcare:* The necessities involved in smart healthcare can be primarily categorized into functional and nonfunctional necessities:
  - Functional necessities fulfill specific needs in the smart healthcare architecture.
  - The nonfunctional necessities in a healthcare system are those attributes on which perception of the healthcare system quality depends (Fig. 9.2).
- *Technologies used to deploy smart healthcare:* Perceptions of smart healthcare vary among scientists and businesses experts, and technological standards apply to every single component of it. The constituents of a smart healthcare structure can be categorized as sensors, actuators, computing hardware, data storage elements and network components.

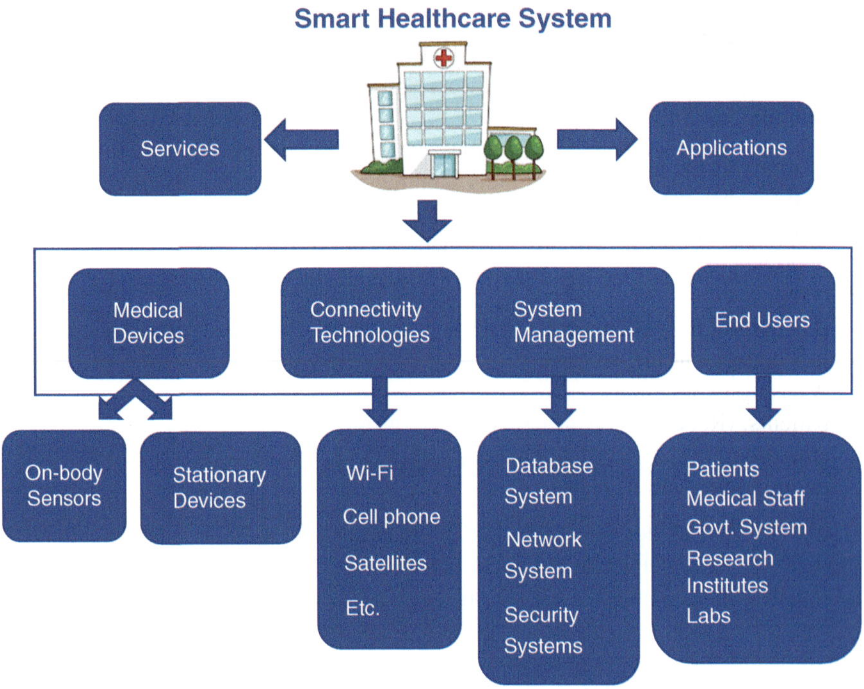

Fig. 9.1 Classification of a smart healthcare system. *Govt.* government

Fig. 9.2 Attributes of smart healthcare

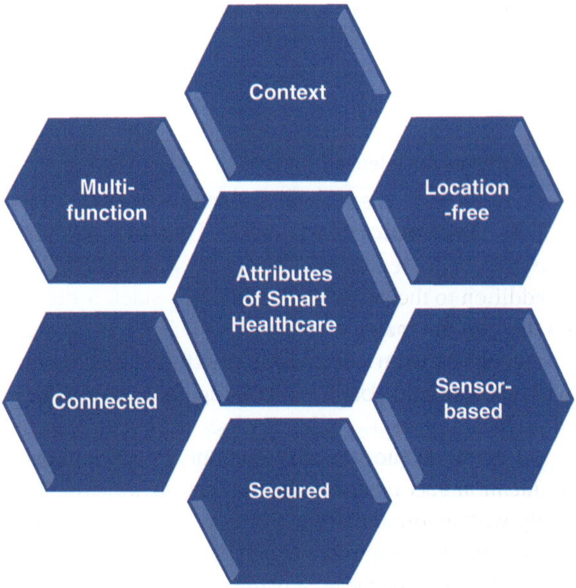

- *Services and applications:* Major services can be provided by different applications in smart healthcare. The services need to be secure, reliable and easily accessible to patients and healthcare professionals [10]. These applications can be classified into three main categories: healthy living, home care and acute care:

1. Healthy living
   a. Health tracking
   b. Disease prevention
   c. Nutritional monitoring
2. Home care:
   a. Mobile health
   b. Telemedicine
   c. Self-care and management
   d. Assisted living
3. Acute Care
   a. Hospital care
   b. Speciality clinic care
   c. Nursing home care
   d. Community hospital care

9.5 Security Requirements of Smart Healthcare

Smart healthcare offers improved healthcare to all members of society but at the same time can be more susceptible to risks and threats. Because of its dynamic nature and reduced form factors, the security requirements and concerns in smart healthcare differ from those in traditional healthcare [11] (Fig. 9.3).

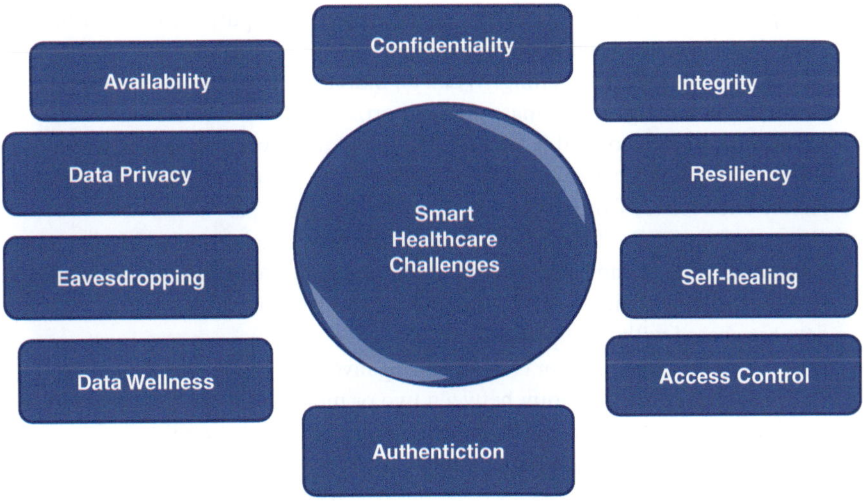

Fig. 9.3 Security requirements and concerns in smart healthcare

The importance of each security requirement in smart healthcare is detailed below [12]:

- *Service availability:* Accessibility ensures that healthcare services and data are accessible to the relevant users when needed by them. Among the most common causes of a denial of service is hacking of access to information, organizations, hardware devices or supplementary networks.
- *Data confidentiality:* This requires fortification of healthcare information to prevent any accidental, illegitimate or unsanctioned access, disclosure or theft. It also requires appropriate measures to ensure that only approved viewing, sharing and use of data can occur.
- *Integrity:* This concerns the accuracy and completeness of the information. The data should remain unchanged during its storage and transfer, and preventive actions should be taken to ensure that the information is not altered by any individual without appropriate authorization.
- *Location confidentiality:* Site discretion defends the location of individuals by changing the conforming information instead of minimizing the site information accuracy.
- *Authentication:* Substantiation involves identifying an individual's uniqueness. Authorizations given by individuals are stored in a file in the databank of accredited users. This information is stored in a validation server.
- *Self-healing:* Ideally, smart healthcare systems should be capable of reverting themselves to their normal state when required. Integration of risk recognition, machine learning and behaviour examination helps in recognizing threats and neutralizing them in a proactive manner.
- *Access control:* This safety practice is responsible for regulating which individuals are authorized to handle the data in a computing setting. It is a vital component in data safety and reduces risk in any kind of business.
- *Exceptional credentials:* The basic requirement for the purpose of identification (ID) checking is possession of an exclusive form of ID verification. This needs to be unique to the specific setting. When an individual is recognized via their user ID, their data access is automatically authorized.
- *Resiliency:* This involve the capability to adapt to varying circumstances and to resist or quickly recover from interruptions. Flexibility includes the ability to handle and recover from deliberate or accidental mishaps.
- *Data confidentiality:* This is part of data security, which is responsible for appropriate data control and management of all necessary controlling responsibilities. It concerns the practical aspects of data confidentiality in terms of how and when data are shared with third parties.
- *Data snooping:* Snooping or eavesdropping involves obtaining information from a confidential communication between two or more parties without them knowing that their communication has been intercepted. Eavesdropping is frequently used to capture private communication.

- *Identity threats:* These are also known as *identity fraud*, which is a criminality offence in which critical information or personal identifiable information (PII) is obtained by a third party who could use it with malicious intent.
- *Data cleanness:* This assumes that data collected by sensors or actuators are up to date and not repeats of older communications.

9.6 Major Risks Related to Smart Healthcare

1. Ethical problems
2. Risks from information leakage
3. Cyber risks
4. Authentication and interoperability issues
5. Health information exchange barriers
6. Health Device communications
7. Management of real-time data

9.7 Security Solution of Smart Health Applications

Confidentiality is one of the prime prerequisites of smart healthcare. Private and personal information on individuals should be shared only among authorized personnel in order to maintain its credibility. Only approved nodes and users should have access to services or resources [12]. To ensure data safety, two-level authentication must be applied to authenticate peer identity. It is vital to maintain integrity in a healthcare network to assure users that any data being transmitted or received remain uncompromised. If, by chance, an interconnected hardware device is compromised, the security system must guarantee the safety of all information on that device and in the healthcare network. Interconnected devices must possess the property of self-healing to prevent adverse impacts on the healthcare system in the event of sudden device failure [11].

9.8 Smart Health System Services

Smart health system services include the following [13]:

- Evidence-based care
- Self-learning and self-improvement
- Big data for real-time data management
- Healthcare IoT applications
- Privacy and security
- Smart employee management

- mHealth devices and apps
- Patient-centred care
- Personalized management
- Operating cost optimization
- Disease management
- Drug management
- Remote patient monitoring
- Preventive care
- Assisted living
- Data collection and analytics
- Flexible rural and urban smart healthcare systems

Smart health has totally changed the healthcare system. Smart systems are continuously enhancing the quality of healthcare. The implementation and deployment of smart healthcare technologies bring many benefits and advantages to healthcare and improve the quality of healthcare services. One of the major challenges in a smart healthcare system is evolution in the direction of smart healthcare, which is proceeding with sustained but slow progress [14]. One of the main reasons for this slow pace is that ongoing training of healthcare specialists is needed to keep pace with new advancements. However, it should be easier for younger generations to understand the benefits of smart health. By bridging the gap between scientists and healthcare experts, unresolved research questions and illnesses can be resolved, thereby improving the quality of life of individuals in a smarter way.

This chapter has discussed the values and risks involved in smart healthcare systems, with a focus on continuous improvement. The existing achievements and further potential of smart healthcare systems have the power to revolutionize traditional healthcare systems and replace them with new technological systems to improve health diagnosis, health monitoring and other healthcare practices.

References

1. Sundaravadivel P, Kougianos E, Mohanty SP, Ganapathiraju MK (2017) Everything you wanted to know about smart health care: evaluating the different technologies and components of the Internet of Things for better health. IEEE Consum Electron Mag 7(1):18–28
2. Bogdanova H (2018) Pros and cons of remote patient monitoring. Health IT Outcomes. https://www.healthitoutcomes.com/doc/pros-and-cons-of-remote-patient-monitoring-0001. Accessed
3. Kulkarni DD, Jakkan DA (2019) A survey on smart health care system implemented using Internet of Things. J Commun Eng Innov 5(1):13–20
4. Mold J (2017) Goal-directed health care: redefining health and health care in the era of value-based care. Cureus 9(2):e1043. https://doi.org/10.7759/cureus.1043
5. Yin H, Akmandor AO, Mosenia A, Jha NK (2018) Smart healthcare. Foundations and Trends in Electronic Design Automation 12(4):401–466. https://doi.org/10.1561/1000000054
6. Oueida S, Aloqaily M, Ionescu S (2019) A smart healthcare reward model for resource allocation in smart city. Multimed Tools Appl 78(17):24573–24594. https://doi.org/10.1007/s11042-018-6647-4

7. Algarni A (2019) A survey and classification of security and privacy research in smart healthcare systems. IEEE Access 7:101879–101894. https://doi.org/10.1109/ACCESS.2019.2930962
8. Appelboom G, Camacho E, Abraham ME, Bruce SS, Dumont EL, Zacharia BE, D'Amico R, Slomian J, Reginster JY, Bruyère O, Connolly ES Jr (2014) Smart wearable body sensors for patient self-assessment and monitoring. Arch Public Health 72(1):28. https://doi.org/10.1186/2049-3258-72-28
9. Chang V, Cao Y, Li T, Shi Y, Baudier P (2019) Smart healthcare and ethical issues. In: Proceedings of the 1st international conference on finance, economics, management and IT business, Heraklion, 3–5 May 2019, pp 53–59. https://doi.org/10.5220/0007737200530059
10. Al-Azzam M, Alazzam MB (2019) Smart city and smart-health framework, challenges and opportunities. Int J Adv Comput Sci Appl 10(2):171–176. https://doi.org/10.14569/IJACSA.2019.0100223
11. Zhang M, Raghunathan A, Jha NK (2014) Trustworthiness of medical devices and body area networks. Proc IEEE 102(8):1174–1188. https://doi.org/10.1109/JPROC.2014.2322103
12. Butt SA, Diaz-Martinez JL, Jamal T, Ali A, De-La-Hoz-Franco E, Shoaib M (2019) IoT smart health security threats. In: Proceedings of the 2019 19th international conference on computational science and its applications (ICCSA), St. Petersburg, 1–4 Jul 2019, pp 26–31. https://doi.org/10.1109/ICCSA.2019.000-8
13. Solanas A, Patsakis C, Conti M, Vlachos IS, Ramos V, Falcone F, Postolache O, Perez-Martinez PA, Di Pietro R, Perrea DN, Balleste MA (2014) Smart health: a context-aware health paradigm within smart cities. IEEE Commun Mag 52(8):74–81. https://doi.org/10.1109/MCOM.2014.6871673
14. Ding D, Conti M, Solanas A (2016) A smart health application and its related privacy issues. In: Proceedings of the 2016 smart city security and privacy workshop, Vienna, 11 Apr 2016, pp 1–5. https://doi.org/10.1109/SCSPW.2016.7509558

Challenges, Opportunities and Future Trends in Smart Health

10

Smart technologies have been in existence for years, but most of them are still in the testing phases. Data-oriented gadgets, sensors and technologies create a very personalized, customized and prototype approach to health and well-being. Smart technologies have not featured in the field of healthcare until recently but are now playing a vital role in improving health and quality of life.

Smart health systems consist of various connected Internet of Things (IoT) devices and sensors, which constantly track the health status of the patient. Smart healthcare is based on highly analytical and practical experiments with results-oriented algorithms that have a very high accuracy rate. It is mostly used to detect and diagnose disease, which helps in implementing effective treatment [1]. The results produced by the devices in a smart healthcare system are based on artificial intelligence (AI), machine learning and supervised learning algorithms. The data that are analysed as inputs into the algorithms are stored in the cloud and known as big data. Analysis of more and more data helps to create accurate diagnostics for general treatment.

To maintain this whole system of smart healthcare, there is a requirement for professional supervisors (also known as smart healthcare professionals) who understand the system well, manage the division of the workload and treat patients. Smart health is not restricted to hospitals; it opens up the possibility for everyone to track their own health status at home or anywhere else. There are enormous applications for health monitoring to support smart health systems.

This chapter explores the challenges, opportunities and future trends in smart health that will change and update the traditional healthcare system as needed over time. This is vital because the population is increasing very rapidly and traditional healthcare systems are not fully able to provide fast and efficient diagnostics or treatment. Thus, with the involvement of human supervision, smart health can take the healthcare system to a higher level to support better, more efficient, more reliable and more rapid treatments, which will contribute great value to human life.

A smart health system consists of smart techniques such as IoT, AI, big data, cyberphysical systems, machine learning, blockchains and supervised learning,

S. Vyas, D. Bhargava, *Smart Health Systems*,
https://doi.org/10.1007/978-981-16-4201-2_10

which are essential in the industrial revolution known as Industry 4.0 [1]. IoT has the goal of providing unified incorporation among numerous smart devices. These smart devices, with the help of sensors, process data computation. Sensors permit observations of environmental factors, while the chipsets in actuators activate smart systems to provide physical responses for the user. All of these sensor-based systems offer efficacy in diverse services based on multiple applications areas such as smart healthcare, smart transportation and smart surveillance systems.

Big data and cloud computing offer high-powered resources and computing capabilities to perform various tasks remotely and retrieve results for applications. The new pattern of supervised learning, AI and machine learning provides users with efficient and advanced services, shorter response times and the ability to adapt to user needs. The demand for healthcare applications has been increasing steadily because of the persistent modern intelligent applications of data. The numbers of patients requiring care, the types of analyses that are needed and the response time requirements are continuing to increase. More and more diseases are being diagnosed daily and have a major effect on people's lives. Access to treatment needs to be evaluated by effective comparisons, and, more importantly, health applications need to be implemented using powerful and dynamic frameworks that provide high-quality and effective outcomes [2].

A smart healthcare system is intended to be a blend of traditional healthcare and smart devices embedded with sensors, wearable gadgets that interconnect with smart healthcare centres, smart emergency response systems, ambulances equipped with smart technologies and innovative techniques combining software-based information and communication technologies. The smart healthcare system is a significant development to support ageing populations, who are vulnerable to many chronic diseases, and younger people, who are vulnerable to various types of exploitation and lifestyle diseases. Smart healthcare technologies such as IoT play active roles in prevention of disease and early diagnosis of symptoms of disease. Smart healthcare engineering includes many variations that come with novel challenges for medical administrations, which can be big or small. Specifically, rapid increases in government regulations, new technologies and patient expectations generate an innovative environment in which healthcare is not limited to treating patients. Digital technology is providing a foundation of data for the future of the intelligent healthcare industry. There are also major challenges involved in achieving the goal of customized healthcare. However, healthcare systems focused on generating actual patient-centred, data-driven and deliverable products have a greater chance of leading the changes in health and well-being. The major challenges for providing smart healthcare involve three main key points:

- Most patients need to have consistent monitoring, and their data should be analysed at every opportunity. Thus, the data volumes are so large that their processing requires hardware that has high computational capacity with support from powerful algorithms.
- Hardware with a high processing capacity is costly, which creates large expenses for healthcare systems.

- It is vital to maintain the integrity and consistency of the system. Healthcare information is very sensitive because it can easily be misused by unauthorized people to target groups of people. It is therefore necessary to have a tamper-proof and secure framework that can keep highly sensitive healthcare data completely secure.

The most important challenge is the need for the capacity to integrate all of the relevant technologies to provide solutions that meet all possible requirements in smart healthcare systems.

10.1 Challenges in Adoption of Smart Healthcare Systems

Smart healthcare systems that influence electronic health records (EHRs) and use techniques such as IoT and big data are expected to link patients and providers flawlessly across different healthcare systems. Smart healthcare systems are also being progressively connected via the Internet to various types of medical sensor device technologies that are connected to the human body for live tracking of health status and healthcare monitoring. To keep healthcare affordable and widely available to everyone, simple computerization and efficient management are required. However, smart healthcare computerization is considered one of the most difficult tasks in building smart infrastructure systems.

The smart infrastructure of healthcare systems needs to be developed by utilizing smart technologies such as IoT, big data, cloud computing, machine learning and AI. Such technologies are envisaged to revolutionize future healthcare systems by suggesting possible real-time options on the basis of active intelligence at a comparatively low cost. AI-enabled tools can perform disease diagnosis and assist doctors to perform surgery and other procedures. Smart healthcare technologies offer the promise of better diagnostic tools, better-quality treatment for patients and better services, thereby improving the quality of life for everyone at a lower cost. The plan of action, unresolved problems, major challenges, and future trends in smart health are discussed below.

10.1.1 Collection or Gathering Information

Collection of data is very important in smart healthcare systems. The density of the data is increasing so quickly that it is becoming very difficult to estimate the data volumes involved. It is difficult to gather data that are context dependent and personalized in participatory scenarios, and the processes that are involved pose major challenges in ensuring reliability, energy efficiency, cost containment, nonintrusiveness and integrability [2]. There are multiple ways to collect data:

- *Sensors embedded in regular mobile devices:* These devices can be attached to the body as wearables or can be other mobile devices that are placed at a precise distance from the body and can take the input responses from the body and track the health status of the body continuously.

- *Radiofrequency waves in impenetrable environments:* Remote wireless monitoring of the patient can be done, and data can be collected with the help of different digital devices, but communication channels can interfere with the quality of the data. An extensive variability about dissimilar and heterogeneous communication arrangements needs to have a parallel existence [3] and could decrease interference and optimize use of propagation channels. It is essential to render it in every scenario. In the case of truly wireless arrangements, interference control plays a vital role in the operation and efficiency of the network. These wireless systems range from very minimal or short ranges (which can be generalized as wireless area networks) to coast-to-coast mobile networks, which work in a very efficient way [4]. Data collection using radiofrequency waves is directly affected by interference in the air medium, but data can be collected wirelessly from frequency-based receivers for real-time patient monitoring.
- *Network-based platforms such as IoT:* IoT plays a vital role in collection of data related to the smart healthcare system. Most devices in a smart healthcare system are IoT based. Devices that are used only for medical and smart healthcare are known as the Internet of Medical Things (IoMT) in smart health. These devices track the real-time status of patients independently.

10.1.2 Storage and Recovery of Data

Storage of data is a crucial element in smart healthcare systems, and they must be kept secure. The massive volumes of big data emphasis on traditional data storage to enhance needs related to scalability and also simplifying the data transformation in the knowledge-base about smart healthcare.

- *New storage techniques:* An interactive database with smart approaches works well with massive volumes of the smart healthcare data. Also, the effective responses about the data analysis delivers in less time. The revolution in the volumes of data now being collected has prompted creation of new storage models such as NoSQL databases, with optimization of efficiency and scalability to read/write huge data volumes, but at the cost of consistency in the storage of the data [2]. There are many other solutions, such as Spark, which offer faster and efficient memory-oriented substitutes for parallel and distributed algorithms in a cluster, and some solutions are ahead in the drive for domains in smart healthcare that use big data processing for storage [5].
- *Formatting and indexing of data:* Formatting and indexing of massive volumes of data are essential attributes of big data and are having substantial impacts on information collection and abstraction processes. Smart healthcare information that is stored in a structured format is more scalable and less time intensive to handle than unstructured information.

10.1.3 Knowledge Acquisition

After collection and storage of the data, it is very important to analyse it and put it into the required format so it can be utilized for its purpose. One approach that is being selected and tested is the recommender systems approach with process mining and deep learning, representing areas of study that will play important roles in smart healthcare in the future [2].

- *Recommender systems:* These types of systems are designed to help the smart healthcare system filter the data for noise and disruptions that have occurred during the transmission of the data.
- *Crowdsourcing systems:* In these systems, massive groups of smart healthcare gadgets and sensors that are capable of sensing and computing (such as smartphones, tablet computers and wearables) supportively share data and abstraction about the information to measure, map, analyse, estimate or make predictions [6].
- *Data mining for smart health:* After successful storage of data, it is very important to have proper data sets available for treatment. More accurate healthcare data can increase the effectiveness and the efficiency of treatment.
- *Deep learning:* Deep learning delivers a smart healthcare system with the capability to analyse data with extraordinary responsiveness without compromising its accuracy. Deep learning in smart healthcare is a blend of both machine learning and AI, which uses layered algorithm architecture to examine the data at an amazing rate. The advantages of deep learning in smart healthcare are that it is fast, well organized, effective and precise.

10.1.4 Smart Healthcare Applications

There are distinct applications for different smart healthcare solutions. The implementation of smart healthcare applications is the final outcome of all of the preceding processes and embodies the solutions to the issues encountered at each step from the data gathering stage onwards [2]. The applications have direct interfaces connecting them to the patient or the user.

10.2 Transformational Challenges for Smart Healthcare Centres

Smart healthcare centre systems have the objective of providing patients and doctors with a platform to provide healthcare services seamlessly and efficiently. Patients can be monitored remotely, and healthcare workers can share real-time information in the event of an emergency [7].

10.2.1 Systems for Patient Monitoring in Smart Healthcare Systems

It is a major challenge to achieve continuous monitoring of patients, delivery of high-quality care, patient safety, supervisory compliance and patient satisfaction in facilities with only small numbers of healthcare staff [8]. This requires effective health monitoring by doctors and alert generation, supported by quick decision-making and prompt responses. Inability to deploy IoT and other technology solutions for patient monitoring are also causes for concern.

10.2.2 Data Accuracy in Smart Healthcare Systems

Machine learning programs are fed information with very high levels of accuracy, but when they learn incorrect patterns, they are likely to provide incorrect insights, resulting in flawed treatment of patients. Thus, there is a need to ensure that only accurate data are fed to the EHR system. There is a chance that data feeds from IoT sensors will not cause problems as long as the sensors are working properly. However, when human beings feed the data, there may be greater chances of error [8].

10.2.3 Cyber-security in Smart Healthcare Systems

Maintaining the confidentiality, integrity and availability of smart healthcare data is a challenge. Storage of healthcare data in nontrusted databases in hospitals is a concern for patients, as there are risks of misuse and tampering with the data. A compromise in the privacy of healthcare data can have major implications in real life. According to the 2017 Cost of Cyber Crime Study by Accenture, the annualized cost of cybercrime in the healthcare industry is US$12.47 million [8]. Cloud storage of healthcare data also causes both security and compliance concerns. According to a 2018 survey by the Symantec Corporation, less secure cloud databases have proven to be vulnerable in various organizations [8].

10.2.4 Reducing the Costs of Devices and Sensors in Smart Healthcare Systems

The growth in the costs of smart healthcare systems' components is a big challenge for patients. Performance and compliance requirements also contribute to hospital costs. There is a trade-off between user convenience and cost. Cloud computing is a way to reduce the start-up expenses involved in EHR implementation. Some hospitals have not implemented EHRs, because of the associated privacy and security issues. However, a hospital cannot become smart without implementing EHRs [8].

10.2.5 Data Processing and Validation in Smart Healthcare Systems

In smart healthcare systems with increased heterogeneity of devices, gadgets, sensors and equipment, the heterogeneity and variety of smart healthcare data also increase. As they contain personal lifestyle data and other diverse health data, validating and extracting useful knowledge from these data becomes very challenging. This can be done only with implementation of AI-based supervised learning algorithms.

10.2.6 Tuning and Interoperability of Smart Healthcare Systems

Operating rooms (ORs) in hospitals are generally crowded with many freestanding devices and supporting systems, with their own interfaces to display data. The smart hospital expectation is that once the physician enters the OR, all screens will be ready with information such as patient data, diagnostic imaging, and preoperative plans projected onto the screens [8]. This is challenging, as many hospitals use different records and systems for storing patient information and some programs may be unable to communicate with each other. Thus, there is a need to integrate all information systems and applications in smart hospitals to allow for display of the relevant patient data. Another challenge relates to IoT sensors' internal operation ability, which refers to the ability to accept and adapt data from different types of IoT sensor devices [8].

10.3 Opportunities in Smart Healthcare

Smart healthcare systems are experiencing a rapid evolution from conventional systems to a disseminated approach to better serve patients [9]. There are two types of technological expansion required for smart healthcare:

1. There is a trend towards transferring a variety of maintenance functions outside the bulwarks of the smart healthcare system by making use of IoT. These techniques allow massive composition of the smart healthcare systems, irrespective of the location of the patient, the worker or the system [10].
2. Machine learning and supervised or different deep learning analytical capabilities are becoming more predominant in smart healthcare.

Thus, in these two important ways, traditional healthcare organizations have started looking into smart technologies. Also, these are the most unexplored parts of the industry but offer immense opportunities for healthcare systems [10]. The technologies of the IoT sensor-based submissions should be anonymous and indispensable for re-defining existence of people in smart healthcare system. IoT designates inspecting gadgets and sensor devices (such as a patient's weighing scales or monitors of blood pressure and blood sugar levels) connected to servers that formulate the data from the physical body for the digital storage medium. They contain data such as sugar levels, blood per unit area, dynamic signs and movement-tracking data. Smart healthcare systems are now using IoT extensively and further developing it to accommodate the requirements of future smart healthcare applications. This creates multiple demands related to heterogeneity of devices, scalability, massive use of wireless data transfer technology, optimal and vital use of energy, data administration, privacy and security, bandwidth flux, data transfer rates, inactivity and delay. In smart healthcare systems, there are particular spots for using numerical technology for the advance patient's responses thus improving functional competence. With the accumulation, smart healthcare systems have ability to integrate back-end and front-end tasks to deliver a trustworthy end-to-end customer-oriented experience. This creates the possibly to shape digital groups for improved provision in operational outcomes, which are able to spread the use of patient information from essential to supplementary systems deep in the smart healthcare network. Changes from traditional to smart healthcare provide the benefits discussed below.

10.3.1 Remote Monitoring

Remote monitoring by healthcare systems in smart homes is anticipated to monitor patients' health status and enable medical advice to be given in the home. It can also enable physicians to diagnose diseases through remote data collection.

10.3.2 Chronic Self-Management

Chronic self-management in smart healthcare is a program that offers self-regulation of chronic diseases in smart homes. The modularity of the system depends on the specific disease, with different requirements for each disease model: a set of specifications for the specific disease and a combination of supporting technologies in the smart home [11].

10.3.3 Performance Improvement

Performance improvement and production are affected by various factors such as health, security, wellness and satisfaction related to the healthcare system.

10.3.4 Behaviour Modification

The changes in the behaviour of the system in dealing with a patient and also the changes in perseverance of the healthcare system modifies the behaviour, and some important changes are [12]:

- Conscious levitation
- Histrionic relief
- Self-evaluation
- Social liberty
- Self-freedom
- Relationship help
- Managing protection
- Controlling stimuli

10.3.5 Detection and Diagnosis

Smart healthcare systems include an advanced, quick and responsive diagnostic system, which includes data mining patterns, AI, machine learning and supervised learning through which healthcare professionals can get a highly accurate idea about disease states and prescribe treatment accordingly.

10.4 Trends Shaping the Future of Smart Healthcare

In smart healthcare systems, the skills that are conveyed in an innovative prototypical model for patient management of data, diagnostics and healthcare distribution are constructive variations. Some features may offset increased medical expenses, obsolete traditional substructure models and incomplete distribution of healthcare amenities in developing and underdeveloped countries. With the increases in demand, patients are becoming more conscious about healthcare problems and want healthier and better services. The main change in healthcare system occurs in many ways, the main reason behind the these changes is consumption of proper healthcare practices among the common people.

Patients seeks for remedial and the medication majorly, and also looks for the effective healthcare procedures. A healthcare service should aim to provide excellence, security and high ethical standards with very reasonable treatment costs, suitability and flexibility. Thus, healthcare systems are changing from a provider-centric model to a customer-centric model. New technologies that combine old analogue technology and newer digital technology are enormously helpful to healthcare systems. With implementation of these novel technologies, some healthcare organizations and governments could easily make progress in improving the health of patients. Healthcare should be less expensive, more easily accessible to people in different sectors of society, more appropriate and more timely. Smart healthcare systems can enable patients to manage themselves in a better way by controlling their own health and medical data [13].

1. *Predictive healthcare:* Predictive analytics facilitates smart healthcare by improving patient care in terms of quality, competence, cost and patient satisfaction.

2. *Virtual care and remote monitoring technology:* Smart healthcare monitoring systems have evolved to facilitate easy operation and ease of communication between healthcare providers and patients for appropriate monitoring, critical health checkups, general consultation and healthy lifestyles [14].
3. *Genomics and gene editing:* In smart healthcare, medicine is experiencing a sector-wide revolution in which advances in networking and computing technologies play vital roles. Healthcare is evolving from a reactive and health-centric model to a prevention and personal practice model—from being disease focused to being health and wellness focused. In short, healthcare systems and basic medical research are progressing intelligently, and significant advances in genomics and genetic engineering are being made with the help of machine learning and AI [15].
4. *Data and AI drives:* Data and AI offer numerous advantages over conventional analytical and decision-making procedures. Machine learning and supervised learning algorithms can be made more accurate as they communicate with trained data sets, allowing people to gain extraordinary insights into diagnoses, care procedures, treatments and patient results.
5. *Big data, IoT and smart cities:* In healthcare, the term *big data* is used to define the vast amount of information generated by implementation of digital technology that gathers patient information and aids management of hospital processes—tasks that are too big and complex for traditional technology. IoT also provides a chance to improve the quality and efficiency of the entire service delivery environment—which includes medical infrastructure management, asset management, staff workflow monitoring and streamlining of medical services—through building of a smart healthcare system based on IoT [16]. New inventions in IoT aid preventive medicine and management of chronic conditions. The aim of smart cities is to improve city structures by minimizing costs, endorsing innovation in different areas and refining the citizens' quality of life.
6. *Telemedicine:* By using these technologies, smart healthcare can efficiently minimize the costs and risks of medical procedures, improve the efficiency of medical facilities, encourage trade and collaboration in various regions, encourage telemedicine and self-care, and, finally, create customized medical services everywhere [17].
7. *AR/VR in healthcare:* Augmented reality (AR) and virtual reality (VR) can be utilized to perform more precise and less risky surgeries and can help surgeons by saving time in emergency surgery. After mining of research papers or electronic medical records (EMRs), all relevant information can be presented on the surgeon's AR screen within seconds.
8. *Blockchain:* Blockchain can handle an entire data system in smart healthcare, where all stakeholders can access the data from a single point safely and securely. Blockchain can have a major impact on the clinical research field in healthcare because they allow for storage, sharing and tracking of data [18].
9. *Applications for tracking healthiness and well-being:* Applications (apps) that track healthiness and well-being deliver abundant profits and are very beneficial for both individual entities and healthcare systems. For example, there

are various systems that can measure the blood pressure, heart rate, sleep duration, distance travelled and number of steps taken with high accuracy. They also allow the data to be viewed in a readable way, store the data, perform statistical analysis, compare results and provide guidance for improving health [13].

10. *Smart infirmaries:* A smart healthcare organization is dependent on a connected structure of smart healthcare gadgets to improve healthcare procedures and introduce innovative new services. The main goal of smart healthcare systems is to change the patient's data into visualized data and then work on those data, utilizing insight. Smart healthcare technologies in smart hospitals focus on collection of precise data and then use data mining with AI, deep learning and machine learning to analyse the data. They then make this information available to medical personnel and other specialists using smart devices such as laptops, tablets, sensor-based devices and smart gadgets.

There is a crucial need to consider using multiple combinations of machine learning and supervised learning techniques to predict setbacks and failures, and to maintain the required level of quality in the data delivered from cloud servers [7]. Integration of health-monitoring applications with different sensors and analytics-based technologies such as AI, supervised learning, VR, robotics, EHRs and telehealthcare systems enables healthcare systems to meet increasing demands and function efficiently to provide excellent and secure healthcare services. A patient can be monitored securely by their own health-monitoring gadgets, with the data being recorded faithfully, accessible to the patient and owned by them, so that their health status and need for doctor's visits are better controlled. In additional ways, this also decreases the load on doctors by allowing them to focus on important matters such as treating more critical conditions, curing illnesses and saving lives. In summary, these new and advanced technologies are now a reality and will continue to transform medicine and health for the better [13]. Numerous efforts are now being made to enhance the quality of healthcare by utilizing fog computing frameworks, with the objective of accurate virus and disease predicting techniques in their respective treatments with automated prescription generation in smart healthcare systems [19].

Smart healthcare systems have the potential to change the whole healthcare system and create a new healthcare environment, which will be based purely on smart things. These improvements in diagnosis and treatment of disease will play a very active role in the world. Minor checkups can possibly be done at home without the need for supervision by a doctor or healthcare professional. With the help of smart IoT devices, healthcare is becoming a much more powerful sector and is empowering people to live healthier lives. Smart healthcare systems are becoming much more robust, reliable and efficient in terms of healthcare data security. Data security is one of the most important aspects of a smart healthcare system; thus, advanced security protocols and analytical algorithms make it more trustworthy to rely upon. The data are kept encrypted during transmission, and there are no loopholes in the security of the data.

This chapter has discussed challenges, opportunities and future trends, and has focused on the continuous improvements that are occurring in healthcare systems. The long-sought achievement and success of these dynamic new smart healthcare systems have the power to transform traditional healthcare systems and replace them with new technological systems to improve diagnosis, health monitoring and other healthcare practices for the benefit of patients.

References

1. Tuli S, Tuli S, Wander G, Wander P, Gill SS, Dustdar S, Sakellariou R, Rana O (2020) Next generation technologies for smart healthcare: challenges, vision, model, trends and future directions. Internet Technol Lett 3(2):e145
2. Solanas A, Casino F, Batista E, Rallo R (2017) Trends and challenges in smart healthcare research: a journey from data to wisdom. In: Proceedings of the 2017 IEEE 3rd international forum on research and technologies for society and industry (RTSI), Modena, 11–13 Sep 2017, pp 1–6. https://doi.org/10.1109/RTSI.2017.8065986
3. Aguirre E, Flores M, Azpilicueta L, López-Iturri P, Falcone F, Ramos V, Solanas A (2014) Implementing context aware scenarios to enable smart health in complex urban environments. In: Proceedings of the 2014 IEEE international symposium on medical measurements and applications (MeMeA), Lisbon, 11–12 Jun 2014, pp 1–4. https://doi.org/10.1109/MeMeA.2014.6860115
4. Lopez-Iturri P, Casino F, Aguirre E, Azpilicueta L, Falcone F, Solanas A (2016) Performance analysis of ZigBee wireless networks for AAL through hybrid ray launching and collaborative filtering. J Sens 2016:2424101. https://doi.org/10.1155/2016/2424101
5. Zhang J, Zhang Y, Hu Q, Tian H, Xing C (2016) A big data analysis platform for healthcare on Apache Spark. In: Proceedings of the 2016 international conference on smart health, Haikou, 24–25 Dec 2016, pp 32–43. https://doi.org/10.1007/978-3-319-59858-1_4
6. Tenney M, Sieber R, Hall GB (2016) Crowd sensing system for public participation. In: International conference on GIScience short paper proceedings. 1 (1). https://doi.org/10.21433/B3116pw0r1dz
7. Rukmani K, Ghankuntla R, Vijay D, Anil T, Adarsh D (2015) Future of wireless technology 6G & 7G. Int J Electr Electron Res 3(2):583–585
8. Ahad A, Tahir M, Yau KLA (2019) 5G-based smart healthcare network: architecture, taxonomy, challenges and future research directions. IEEE Access 7:100747–100762. https://doi.org/10.1109/ACCESS.2019.2930628
9. Chen M, Li W, Hao Y, Qian Y, Humar I (2018) Edge cognitive computing based smart healthcare system. Futur Gener Comput Syst 86:403–411. https://doi.org/10.1016/j.future.2018.03.054
10. SyberScribe (2020) 10 emerging trends in healthcare technology for 2020 and beyond. https://www.syberscribe.com.au/blog/10-emerging-trends-healthcare-technology-2019-beyond/. Accessed on 15/3/2021
11. Teriús-Padrón JG, Kapidis G, Fallmann S, Merdivan E, Hanke S, García-Betances RI, Cabrera-Umpierrez MF. Towards self-management of chronic diseases in smart homes: physical exercise monitoring for chronic obstruction pulmonary disease patients. In: Proceedings of the 2018 IEEE international conference on pervasive computing and communications workshops (PerCom Workshops), Athens, 19–23 Mar 2018, pp 776–781. https://doi.org/10.1109/PERCOMW.2018.8480163
12. Taiwo O, Ezugwu AE (2020) Smart healthcare support for remote patient monitoring during COVID-19 quarantine. Inform Med Unlocked 20:100428
13. Ahmad M, Amin MB, Hussain S, Kang BH, Cheong T, Lee S (2016) Health fog: a novel framework for health and wellness applications. J Supercomput 72(10):3677–3695. https://doi.org/10.1007/s11227-016-1634-x

14. Zhao W, Luo X, Qiu T (2017) Smart healthcare. Appl Sci 7(11):1176. https://doi.org/10.3390/app7111176
15. Kelly JT, Campbell KL, Gong E, Scuffham P (2020) The Internet of Things: impact and implications for health care delivery. J Med Internet Res 22(11):e20135
16. Tian S, Yang W, Le Grange JM, Wang P, Huang W, Ye Z (2019) Smart healthcare: making medical care more intelligent. Glob Health J 3(3):62–65
17. Shukla RG, Agarwal A, Shukla S (2020) Blockchain-powered smart healthcare system. In: Krishnan S, Balas VE, Julie EG, Robinson YH, Balaji S, Kumar R (eds) Handbook of research on blockchain technology. Academic, London, pp 245–270
18. Sebastian MP (2019) Smart hospitals: challenges and opportunities., Working paper no. 315. Kozhikode, Indian Institute of Management Kozhikode
19. Ahmed SM, Rajput A (2020) Chapter 16—threats to patients' privacy in smart healthcare environment. In: Lytras MD, Sarirete A (eds) Innovation in health informatics. Academic, London, pp 375–393. https://doi.org/10.1016/B978-0-12-819043-2.00016-2

GPSR Compliance

The European Union's (EU) General Product Safety Regulation (GPSR) is a set of rules that requires consumer products to be safe and our obligations to ensure this.

If you have any concerns about our products, you can contact us on ProductSafety@springernature.com

In case Publisher is established outside the EU, the EU authorized representative is:

Springer Nature Customer Service Center GmbH
Europaplatz 3
69115 Heidelberg, Germany

Batch number: 10732044

Printed by Printforce, the Netherlands